Sex
Herbs

Sex Herbs

NATURE'S SEXUAL ENHANCERS FOR MEN AND WOMEN

BETH ANN PETRO ROYBAL
GAYLE SKOWRONSKI

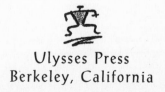

Ulysses Press
Berkeley, California

Published by: Ulysses Press
P.O. Box 3440
Berkeley, CA 94703-3440

Library of Congress Catalog Card Number: 99-60325
ISBN: 1-56975-185-4

Printed in Canada by Transcontinental Printing

10 9 8 7 6 5 4 3 2 1

Editor: Mark Woodworth
Cover Design: Sara Glaser, Leslie Henriques, Sarah Levin
Cover Illustration: "A Day in the Meadow," Hyacinth
    Manning/SuperStock Fine Arts
Herb illustrations are by QuickArt®, copyright by Wheeler Arts
Editorial and production staff: Lily Chou, David Wells
Indexer: Sayre Van Young

Distributed in the United States by Publishers Group West, in Canada by Raincoast Books, and in Great Britain and Europe by Airlift Book Company.

This book has been written and published strictly for informational purposes, and in no way should it be used as a substitute for consultation with your medical doctor or health care professional. All facts in this book came from medical files, clinical journals, scientific publications, personal interviews, published trade books, self-published materials by experts, magazine articles, and the personal-practice experiences of the authorities quoted or sources cited. You should not consider educational material herein to be the practice of medicine or to replace consultation with a physician or other medical practitioner. The author and publisher are providing you with information in this work so that you can have the knowledge and can choose, at your own risk, to act on that knowledge. The author and publisher also urge all readers to be aware of their health status and to consult health professionals before beginning any health program, including changes in dietary habits.

Table of Contents

Note from the authors

For each herb, we'll describe what it does, give some history about its use, and mention which parts of the plant are used. Then we'll describe the sex benefits associated with the herb as well as how to find and use the herb. If the plant's chemical makeup has been determined or active ingredients have been isolated, we'll list them. We'll also mention any cautions or side effects.

You will probably notice that some herbs are listed in more than one chapter. This is because many herbs affect several aspects of sexuality. Saw palmetto, for instance, can help with sexual drive as well as with impotence.

A NOTE ABOUT FORMS OF HERBS Unless noted otherwise, these herbs can be found in pill or extract form. Follow the instructions for dosage on the label of each product.

PART I

THE WONDERFUL WORLD OF HERBS

As long as plants and people have coexisted, we have looked for ways to use plants to better our lives—including our sex lives. And for good reason. One recent study shows that 31 percent of men and 43 percent of women have sexual problems! If a few dried-up leaves or roots can help make sex more pleasurable, it only makes sense to give it a try. The advent of "scientific research" into sexuality has made herbs less popular up until recently. But these days, it seems that practically everyone is trying some herb to enhance their sex lives. Maybe it's time for you to give it a try, too!

Chapter 1 describes what herbs are and how they've been used throughout time and throughout the world. Chapter 2 describes how to choose and use herbs, including information about various forms you'll find herbs in and how to store them to maximize potency.

What Is an Herb?

What do you think of when you hear the word "herb"? A contented cow munching on grass? All those Latin plant names you had to memorize in high school? Your Aunt Lucy's secret recipe for pasta sauce? A New-Age vegetarian type snipping little green things from the pots lined up outside the back of an old VW bus?

A Simple Definition

"Herb" is one of those words that conjures up a variety of unusual images in our minds. Yet, the definition is actually straightforward: An herb is any part of any plant that humans find a personal use for, such as cooking, flavoring, medicine, aroma, or bathing. In fact, the term "herb" is slowly giving away to a more inclusive and perhaps better understood word: "botanical." So, that container of shampoo or body lotion you bought last week with the term "botan-

> *Herb (pronounced urb): Any part of any plant for which humans find a personal use.*

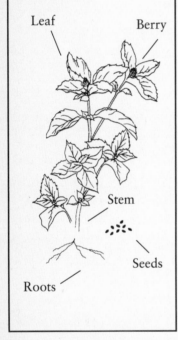

Leaf

Berry

Stem

Seeds

Roots

ical" as part of its name simply contains herbs—or plants (though it likely contains other products as well).

Discovering the Uses of Herbs

The part of the plant used as an herb or botanical could be the leaf, stem, flower, root, bark, berry, or seed. Different parts of even the same plant can have wildly different effects. Some roots, for example, may be deadly, while the leaf of the same plant may be harmless. Some herbs can only be used externally, while others can be safely eaten.

Given all these variables, can you imagine how painstaking it must have been for the ancients to begin sorting through the various uses for herbs? Despite the difficulties, the effort to understand the role of herbs can be seen throughout history all over the world. Perhaps that's one reason why the role of healer has been revered everywhere. Whatever the title—"healer," "medicine woman," "shaman," *curadero*, "herbalist," and more—these people were, and in many regions still are, responsible for knowing (among other things) the appropriate uses of hundreds or even thousands of local herbs.

Ironically, today in our "small world" we are in the enviable position of being able to benefit from herbs grown all over. Yet, many of us are less likely than our ancestors to use this knowledge to enhance our health and well-being, deferring instead to what we now call "traditional Western medicine." The reason? There are many. But perhaps the most important and most relevant for this book is our reliance on "scientific method" to prove the safety and effectiveness of any given therapy.

Measuring the Effectiveness of Herbs

The big question remains: Can herbs improve your sex life? Millions of people throughout the ages would say, "Absolutely!" Many physicians would say, "Probably not, except in a few circumstances." Why the widely diverging opinions? And what should you think— and do—with such conflicting stories?

In our society today, there are two basic ways to assess the effectiveness of any substance or treatment, be it herb or medicine: these are the scientific method and anecdotal evidence. Researchers following the scientific method carefully design studies to control other variables that could affect the results. So, for example, if scientists were investigating a new medication, several steps would be followed:

Testing on animals to see if the treatment has any effect.

Testing on a few humans, usually people who are extremely ill or who have tried every other therapy to no avail. This helps establish the range of doses that are effective without being toxic.

"Double-blind" testing with a larger group of people who could potentially benefit from the therapy. One group receives the test therapy, while the other group receives a placebo (such as a "sugar pill") that will not affect them—or receives no treatment at all. Ideally, neither the patients nor those involved in the study know who is receiving which treatment, hence the term double-blind. Testing usually runs for several years. Results between the two groups are then compared.

For medications and other therapies, once the study is completed, the researchers apply to the U.S. Food and Drug Administration for approval to market the product or therapy. The application includes all test results and any noted side effects. The FDA can take years to review the results, request additional studies, and make a decision.

As you can see, this research process is lengthy and expensive. And the payoff is not guaranteed—after all, herbs cannot be patented, unlike prescription drugs. Any research one company would conduct to prove the usefulness of its herb could easily prove the usefulness of the competitor's herb as well. An herbal product can only be patented if an active ingredient is extracted and formulated into a separate product. Yet, if a company pursues this route, they must follow all the FDA requirements for investigating a new medication. The process and cost involved in this type of research put it beyond the reach of most companies that market herbal preparations. In fact, one company that was trying to develop medicines based on herbs discovered in rainforests just gave up, stating that the FDA process was both too expensive and cumbersome. Instead, it is forming a new subsidiary to market herbal supplements and other herbal products, for which there are no FDA requirements.

The lack of detailed research about the efficacy of an herb forces us either to ignore the possible benefits that come from using herbs or to rely on another type of research: anecdotal evidence. Anecdotes are simply individual reports of a person's experience with an herb. As anecdotes collect over time, you can often begin to see patterns in what works, and how. This is the way the effectiveness of herbs has been "documented" throughout the ages. However, this method isn't foolproof. For example, if you began taking

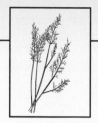

Did You Know?

Many pharmaceutical researchers focus on identifying plants with medicinal properties. Traditionally, research for these plants—called phytopharmaceuticals (phyto meaning to ward off or protect)—has been spearheaded by university schools of pharmacy or government researchers. However, the giant pharmaceutical companies are increasingly conducting phytopharmaceutical research themselves, in hopes of identifying their next highly profitable breakthrough drugs.

an herb to increase your sexual pleasure, it may be difficult to tell whether a positive effect came from the herb itself or from some other factor, such as adjusting blood pressure medication or practicing meditation to relieve stress or simply being hopeful that you can make an important change in your life.

It's this lack of "control" over the research that leads many physicians and patients to discount herbal therapies until they have been "proven" scientifically. Nonetheless, anecdotes do provide at least a general indication of what works—and it's the primary type of research relied on in this book.

So what should you make of this? First, remember that most of us are looking for herbs to enhance sex, not to treat a serious health condition. For this purpose, as long as you use caution, you're unlikely to be hurt and may find benefits from using herbs. It will probably take some time and experimentation, however, to discover the combination of herbs that works best for your needs.

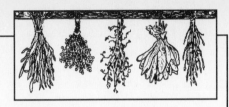

Did You Know?

As much as 75 percent of all patented medications are derived from herbs. One example is digoxin, which is the primary ingredient for many drugs manufactured to treat heart disease. You may be interested to know that digoxin is derived from leaves from the common foxglove plant. (But don't eat foxglove on your own! Foxglove is considered highly poisonous.)

For folks who have serious health problems that in some way inhibit sex, you'll want to use even more caution, keep your healthcare team informed about any herbs you use, and consider consulting with someone who understands herbs. Many "traditional" physicians and nurses are taking the time to learn more about herbs and other "alternative" therapies. Also, herbalists, naturopaths, acupuncturists, chiropractors, and other alternative healthcare practitioners can provide valuable assistance. Look for someone who has had professional training and is certified in herbal medicine.

2

How to Choose and Use Herbs

So if you want to try using an herb described in this book, do you just head out to the nearby field and pull up something that looks like the herb? Probably not. This chapter explains the many forms herbs take, how to select and store herbs, whom to consult when you need more information or advice about particular herbs or particular sex concerns, how herbs interact with other herbs and medications, and the role of herbs in your greater plan for maintaining your health.

The Many Forms of Herbs

When we describe a particular herb in this book, we'll give you information on the various forms in which the herb can be safely used. Using the herb in the wrong way may render it ineffective—or perhaps even downright dangerous. Following are descriptions of some of the forms in which herbs are typically used. Throughout the book you may also find special references to unique herbal products that do not fit these categories, such as herbal beverages, creams, or even soft drinks.

Fresh herbs   Many herbs can be used fresh. These are most effective if grown in your own garden. When they are harvested can alter their potency—there is generally a "best time" to pick most herbs. Other factors affecting potency include soil, as well as exposure to light, heat, and oxygen during storage and transportation.

Pay close attention to which part of the herb should be used: root, stem, leaf, flower, seed, berry, and so on. Pay even closer attention to any parts that should *not* be used! Fresh herbs may be used whole or crushed or chopped. Often, fresh herbs are added to salads, sauces, or other food; infused in teas; placed in bathwater; or used in potpourri. Fresh herbs are generally sold by herb shops, health food stores, and, to some extent, grocery stores.

When Growing Your Own...

Some herbalists recommend against using homegrown herbs for medicinal purposes. Their concern is that you have no way to ensure consistent levels of the active ingredients. Others, however, feel that since most herbs used from the home garden aren't usually needed in great quantities, there is little risk of toxicity and there are few long-term ramifications if the "dose" is less than therapeutic.

Dried herbs   You can grow and dry your own herbs or purchase them dried. If you use dried herbs, remember that herbs shrink as they dry, so you'll need less than you would for fresh herbs. Sources for dried herbs range from your local supermarket, to health food stores, to herb shops, to providers of herbal medical services, to ethnic herbal medicine stores. Dried herbs are also often powdered and may be formed into pills. You can even find combinations of herbs in pill form, many marketed with sexy-sounding names to indicate their purpose. These are found at the same sources as above, and through many drugstores and mail order companies.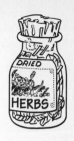

DRYING HOMEGROWN HERBS It's easy to dry fresh herbs. Start with herbs that are free of bug holes and other damage. Then follow these steps.

1. Make sure the herbs are clean. Rinse lightly and gently with water, if needed.

2. You can pick off individual leaves now (assuming the leaf is the part you want to dry), or keep the leaves and stems intact until after they are dried.

3. Arrange the herbs in a single layer on a baking tray.

4. Place the herbs in a sunny location protected from wind and insects, or dry them in the oven at about 100°F or less. The amount of time it takes to dry them depends on how much moisture they were holding to begin with and the temperature and humidity of the location in which they are drying. It may take a few hours or a few days.

5. When the herbs are completely dried out, if you have not already done so, remove the leaves from the stems. Simply roll the stems between your palms and the dried leaves will fall, crushed.

6. Store the herbs in an airtight container.

Tea or infusion   Many times herbs are infused or soaked in water or another liquid. The resulting tea is then strained and used either as a drink or externally as a salve or poultice. Be sure to follow steeping times closely to avoid a substance that is either ineffective or too potent. Many companies also offer herbal teas for internal use. They are available through supermarkets, drugstores, and health food stores.

Poultice or salve   Herbs or herbal infusions can be mixed with other substances to form thicker poultices or salves for external use. Often you can make your own. Or many types of herbal salves are available through drugstores and health food stores.

Extraction or tincture   Often a concentrated form of an herb is required. To create the concentration, the herb is steeped in alcohol, water, oil, or other liquid. It may then be strained. Extractions can sometimes be made at home. It is often easier to purchase them at health food stores and through herbalists or ethnic herb shops. Extractions may be taken internally, used externally, or used for aromatherapy. Most extractions are in alcohol. However, it is possible to find some extractions that are water-based or oil-based. Most extractions are used as drops to be placed on the back of the tongue. Some extractions come in small spray cans.

Oils and essences   Plants contain two types of oils: volatile and fixed. Volatile oils break down easily, releasing the aroma from the plant. Volatile oil is also called *essence*. Fixed oil does not break down as easily and may be used for other purposes. Plant oils can be used in a variety of ways: internally, externally, or for aromatherapy. Creating oils requires great quantities of the herb, making it more cost- and time-effective to purchase the oil through a drugstore, health food store, herbalist, or herb shop. Oils and essences used for aromatherapy or potpourri can also be found where perfumes and bath products are sold.

Preserving and Storing Your Herbs

In general, it's best to store herbs in a cool, dry, dark place. Different herbal forms may have different storage requirements. An alcohol-based extraction will lose its potency quickly if stored in the light. Some nonalcohol extractions may require refrigeration. Dried herbs probably do not require refrigeration, but should be stored in airtight containers. Fresh herbs should be used immediately, or stored in the refrigerator for up to a few days. Other special storage requirements will be described throughout the book as needed.

Wherever you store your herbs, be sure they are well out of the reach of children and pets. Although poisoning is unlikely, it can occur. Even children who barely qualify as toddlers can easily unscrew the lids to most spice containers, for example.

Tips for Purchasing and Using Herbs

Sometimes buying and using an herb is as simple as finding it on the shelf at your local grocery store and adding a bit of it to a favorite recipe. However, many herbs are used in greater quantities to achieve therapeutic effects or are relatively difficult and expensive to produce. Because the cost can be high, you'll want to be sure you've made the wisest choice for your own needs. Here are some tips to keep in mind when purchasing herbs.

Let the buyer beware! Do you assume that herbal products must be regulated by the U.S. Food and Drug Administration or some other government agency? Guess again. Not only does the FDA lack the resources needed to monitor herbal products, but it also lacks the mandate. A few years back, the U.S. Congress specifically limited the FDA's ability to regulate nutritional supplements, including herbs. Manufacturers of herbal products are supposed to adhere to these guidelines:

Text continued on page 20.

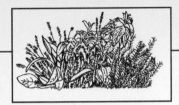

Setting the Mood

Most sex therapists insist that sex begins in your head—in a way, it's an idea that overtakes you. Your body's physical reaction—hormone surges, growing sensitivity of the genital areas, and all the rest—follows. A key part of starting that sexual idea is setting the mood. And herbs can certainly help. The herbs listed below can create the right climate for enjoyable sex, influencing your feelings and mood rather than necessarily changing your body chemistry (though some of these herbs may do that as well). Because what appeals to us and makes us "in the mood" is so individual, view these suggestions as possibilities to get you started.

AROMATHERAPY *Aromatherapy means using scent to evoke a response, such as greater concentration, relaxation, or even putting you in a sexy mood. You can find many oils of aromatic herbs in health food stores and home decorating stores. Or use dried flowers or potpourri placed in a dish. One aroma scientifically proven to evoke feelings of sexuality is the odor of cinnamon buns baking in the oven! The list of herbs whose aromas can create desire for sex is endless and subjective—experiment with scents that appeal to you and your partner. These will get you started: basil, cardamom, cinnamon, jasmine, lavender, patchouli, sandalwood, and vanilla.*

BATHS *One of the best ways to start a romantic encounter is by sharing an herbal bath. Place any combination* of these herbs—dried or fresh—in a cheesecloth bag or tea infuser, letting the herbs soak in warm water along with you. Or try bath oils containing any of these herbs: aloe vera, basil, chamomile, cinnamon, comfrey, eucalyptus, hops, lavender, oats, parsley, and St. John's wort.

BODY PRODUCTS Herbs can help make bodies more appealing by deodorizing them providing aroma, and offering smooth-textured skin. Many body products, such as soap, deodorants, lotions, shampoos, and body oils, have herbs added. Or you can experiment with making your own, from this list of herbs (check for them or their oils at health food stores or herb shops): almond, aloe vera, anise, basil, black and green teas, calendula, chamomile, eucalyptus, jojoba oil, lemon, mugwort, myrrh, oats, olive, pansy, papaya, parsley, sage, and tea tree oil.

BREATH FRESHENERS Essential mood-setters are those delicious kisses that send shivers down the spine. One way to avoid a turn-off from halitosis is to freshen your breath with your own herbal mouth wash. Take several ounces of fresh or dried herbs from the following list, put them in a lidded jar, and fill the jar with vodka. Steep for a few days, then get ready to sip it and pucker up! Herbal breath fresheners include anise, basil, cardamom, cinnamon, clove, coriander, dill, eucalyptus, fennel, ginger, parsley, peppermint, rosemary, sage, spearmint, and turmeric. For parsley, anise, fennel, and the like, eat the greenery or suck on a few seeds to freshen your breath; or try herbs in breath mints or chewing gum.

❖ The product should list all ingredients it contains.

❖ Health claims cannot be made on the labeling. This means that the label will give you very little information about the uses of a given herb or the amount that you should take. It's up to you to find out what each herb does and how much of it is safe to use.

❖ If the product contains nutrients (such as vitamins or minerals) that exceed the **Recommended Dietary Intake (RDI—** formerly called the RDA or Recommended Daily Allowance) per dose, then the amount of the nutrients must be listed.

However, the FDA doesn't routinely follow up with herbal manufacturers to make sure they are complying with these guidelines. In fact, the FDA generally responds to a given herbal product only when problems or serious complaints arise. Otherwise it is assumed that manufacturers are truthful in their product descriptions and claims. Some studies indicate that this assumption may be unfounded, because many nutritional supplements that have been analyzed—including herbal products—contained little (if any!) of the stated ingredients and contained many other ingredients that were unlisted. To find out whether any FDA warnings exist for herbal products, you can contact the FDA (see "Resources" for more information).

Choose a reputable source. Short of opening up your own analytical lab, it's difficult to be sure that any products you purchase are really what they say they are. The best way to ensure high-quality herbal products is to purchase them from a reputable vendor who acquires them from well-known manufacturers. There have been many reports of people finding out that the herbal product they bought contains little or none of the herb listed on the label. Look for companies that guarantee their products' contents in writing.

Common Sources of Herbal Products

❖ Grocery stores
❖ Health food or nutritional supplement stores
❖ Drugstores
❖ Mail order and Internet companies
❖ Independent distributors or sales agents
❖ Specialty stores (such as Chinese herb shops or bath and body products stores)
❖ Alternative healthcare providers
❖ Traditional healthcare providers

Use your resources. Perhaps the best way to ensure wise use of herbs is to talk to people who know about herbs. Gradually, some physicians and nurses are becoming familiar with the more common herbs or herbs that are touted for specific health conditions, such as St. John's wort for depression. Some may even offer herbs for sale through their office (but check elsewhere first—you may be able to find the same herb for less money). A number of medical schools now offer programs in alternative medicine, such as Stanford University's Alternative and Complementary Medicine Program. But at this time you're probably more likely to get good information about herbs from other sources.

Perhaps the best source of accurate information about the use of herbs is from someone who has received formal training in herbal medicine—even if you're not suffering from a particular health condition but simply want to use herbs to enhance your enjoyment of sex. Practitioners of herbal medicine may include any of the following:

❖ Herbalists, who focus solely on the use of plants for medicinal purposes

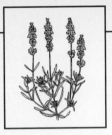

You Know Things Have Changed When...

At least one major health insurance plan—Blue Cross—has formed a partnership with a nutritional supplements company to offer high-quality vitamins and herbs (with guaranteed content) at heavily discounted prices to Blue Cross members. Blue Cross does not cover the cost of herbal preparations, as it would with prescription medicines. However, its willingness to provide inexpensive access to herbal preparations shows how much more respect herbal therapies are receiving today.

❖ Naturopaths, who combine several "natural" therapies to treat health conditions

❖ Acupuncturists, who often use herbal therapies in conjunction with acupuncture

❖ Other certified practitioners of alternative medicine, such as practitioners of Chinese medicine or Ayurvedic medicine (a medical tradition that originated in India), who often use herbs in their therapies

These practitioners may prescribe herbs for a range of health conditions. Often they have advanced academic degrees, such as a master's degree or doctorate in plant biology, in addition to certification from a school of alternative medicine. Check to be sure that whoever you consult with is certified through the appropriate school or association. Ask for references you can contact. You may not even need a one-to-one consultation; many herbalists offer occasional seminars on herbal medicine. Check "alternative" newspapers, local publications, and notices on bulletin boards at health food stores.

You may also find a wealth of information about herbs and their uses from persons with degrees in plant biology or pharmacology. The U.S. Government's Department of Agriculture, for example, has employed plant biologists to search for plants with medicinal and other "practical" uses that could be grown in the United States. Many schools of pharmacy and departments of biology within universities have faculty who have specialized in this area, as well.

Finally, ask the staff at any health food or nutritional supplement stores in your area. People who work in these positions usually have a passion for living "naturally" and may be quite knowledgeable about herbs and their uses. They can also be helpful in recommending brands and other resources.

Whom to Consult About Herbs

❖ Traditional healthcare practitioners, such as doctors (M.D.s or D.O.s), dietitians or nutritionists, and nurses
❖ Herbalists
❖ Naturopaths
❖ Acupuncturists
❖ Other "alternative" health practitioners
❖ Persons with advanced degrees in plant biology
❖ Persons with advanced degrees in pharmacology
❖ Health food store staff

Watch out for side effects. Swallowing a few leaves or drinking a tea made from a plant seems so benign. But herbs can have potent effects. Depending on your sensitivity to particular herbs and the quantities used, many herbs can cause unwelcome effects ranging from flu-like symptoms, to gastrointestinal problems, to liver problems, and even death. In addition, some herbs can make other herbs and medications more potent. For instance, St. John's wort can cause antianxiety medications to act more strongly in the body, even leading to coma. And you may be surprised to find out that certain herbs such as kava can become addictive, much like alcohol, street drugs, or prescription narcotics.

If you notice any unusual effects after taking an herb, discontinue use. Consult with your doctor or a qualified herbalist or other practitioner familiar with herbs. Whomever you consult with, be sure you describe which herbs you have used, the quantities used, and for how long. You may not need to permanently discontinue use of the herb, but may need a smaller quantity of the herb or of other medications that it interacts with.

The Blending of Traditional and Alternative Therapies

Health plans paying for acupuncture . . . Medical doctors taking coursework in herbal therapy . . . Dietitians becoming well-versed in the role of nutritional supplements . . . Pharmaceutical companies buying up herb companies . . . One-A-Day and Centrum introducing new lines of herbal supplements tailored for persons of both sexes and a range of ages . . . These recent changes in traditional medicine and related industries may seem inconsequential; however, when you realize the disdain with which traditional healthcare practitioners and pharmaceutical companies viewed alternative therapies for so long, these changes are truly revolutionary. Some of these shifts in philosophy and practice may have resulted from the incredible profits to be made from a booming market in herbal and other nutritional supplements. But at least some of these changes are linked to the ever-growing emphasis on wellness, versus simply curing illness.

Whatever the cause for these new directions in traditional medicine, you can benefit from the results. Knowledge about herbs and their role in improving sex is growing rapidly as healthcare workers, alternative healthcare practitioners, and researchers all gather more information and experience in this area. The good news is that you can now draw on the resources of both traditional medicine and herbal medicine to achieve the best sex possible.

PART II

HERBS TO IMPROVE YOUR SEX LIFE

How do herbs help with sex? The term "aphrodisiac" probably comes to mind right away. An aphrodisiac (the word derives from *Aphrodite*, the Greek goddess of love and beauty) is anything that provokes sexual interest or desire. And it's true—many herbs can enhance sexual desire. But when it comes to sex, herbs can do more than that. They can:

- Set the mood
- Increase sexual desire and drive (see Chapter 3)
- Increase sexual pleasure (see Chapter 4)

Furthermore, herbs can also aid health conditions that might otherwise inhibit sex. These conditions include the following:

- The "male" problems of impotence, prostate problems, and male menopause (see Chapter 5)

- The "female" problems of menopause and premenstrual syndrome (see Chapter 6)
- Chronic health problems such as arthritis or diabetes (see Chapter 7)
- Other conditions that affect your overall well-being, such as lack of energy or addiction to cigarettes, alcohol, or drugs (see Chapter 8)

In Chapter 9 a brief overview of herbal combinations is offered.

Everyone can probably benefit from reading Chapters 3–4— and Chapters 8 and 9 as well. Chapters 5–7 provide specific information about herbs to aid common health concerns.

3

Increasing Your Sexual Desire and Drive

The word "libido" isn't used now as much as it was in the heyday of Freudian psychology. But its definition still aptly describes "sexual drive." One dictionary puts it this way: "The psychic and emotional energy associated with bodily drives." Another dictionary adds that these "bodily drives" arising from "primitive urges" are usually "goal-oriented." Now, what could *that* mean when we're talking about sex? In this chapter our goal is to focus on sexual desire and drive, which are inextricably connected.

The sexual drive is perhaps the most fascinating of all the "bodily drives." True, its original purpose may have been to ensure the continuation of humankind. But the concept of procreation probably ranks much lower on most of our scales than a desire for plain, "old-fashioned" sexual enjoyment.

But if you don't have the urge—the libido or desire or drive—then you may not be having sex as often as you would like. Or, lack of sexual drive can turn sex into more of a chore than a pleasure. *It doesn't have to be that way.* The herbs described in this chapter can help put sexual desire and drive back into your life—or back into the life of the person you love.

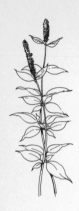

Anise and Star Anise

Pimpinella anisum

Anise is native to the Eastern Mediterranean areas, Eurasia, and Africa. There are approximately 150 different species of anise. All are notable for their feathery leaves and small white or yellow flowers, as well as their licorice-like aroma and taste.

The basics of anise

Anise has a wonderfully rich history—and a significant one, it appears, as it is considered to be one of the oldest medicinal herbs. In biblical times, anise was actually one of the spices that folks used to pay their taxes. The Romans also found good uses for anise, including eating spice cake that included anise as one of its main ingredients. This cake was eaten after a meal to promote good digestion and eliminate indigestion.

Anise is still an extremely popular herb, not only for medicinal purposes, but also for its wide use as a flavoring agent or spice. It is often found in commercially prepared cough medications and throat lozenges. It is also used as an antiseptic in some brands of mouthwash and toothpaste.

It has been shown that many women with a higher level of female sex hormones experience increased sexual desire or even more profound heights of sexual intensity and satisfaction. Anise imitates the female hormone, estrogen. This may explain why anise has been used as a sexual stimulant for women. There are reports, too, that some men using anise have experienced a more satisfying

New Mexican Pumpkin Bread

This has always been a Roybal family favorite. Maybe now we understand why! This recipe produces four loaves of mildly sweet bread. Try it toasted with butter for a satisfying treat or side dish.

7 cups all-purpose flour	*¾–1 cup pumpkin (canned*
1 tablespoon salt	*or fresh cooked)*
⅔ cup sugar	*· 1 tablespoon anise seed*
¼ cup oil	*¾ cups warm water*
2 eggs	*2 packages of yeast*

Mix flour, salt, and sugar. Cut in oil. Beat eggs slightly and add. Add pumpkin. Dissolve yeast in water and add to mixture. Add anise seed. The bread dough will be somewhat sticky—don't add in extra flour unless it's actually soggy.

Let rise two hours. Punch down and knead slightly. Let rise 45 minutes. Punch down, shape, and place in oiled pans. Let rise until doubled in bulk. Bake at 400°F for 20–35 minutes. Check frequently after 20 minutes. It's done when the top is slightly browned and the loaf sounds hollow when tapped.

too, that some men using anise have experienced a more satisfying sex life.

Anise itself has not been formally studied for its effects on sexual stimulation. However, it is generally accepted that anethole, an ingredient of anise, does have mild estrogenic effects.

Parts used

The fruit (seeds) of the anise plant are used for medicinal purposes.

Chemical content

Anise is high in anethole, a compound with effects similar to estrogen, a female sex hormone.

Dosing instructions and availability

Anise seeds are readily available in the spice sections of grocery stores. You may also find it as an ingredient in many food products. You can even find it in some herbal teas. The liqueur anisette also contains anise. The best way to use anise is to add it to recipes for baked goods and desserts. Anise oil is also available. Follow the labeling instructions carefully.

Cautions

Anise is considered safe when used for food. Anise oil can cause vomiting and seizures, so limit use to less than a teaspoon per day. Pregnant women should limit anise to food use only, since its estrogenic effects could cause uterine contractions. Allergic reactions to anethole include redness and blistering with topical use or gastrointestinal distress when anise is eaten.

Added benefits

- May aid iron absorption
- Relieves painful flatulence
- Aids digestion
- Eases respiratory conditions, including asthma and sinusitis, by helping the body to clear mucus from airways
- Repels insects
- Helps to relieve menopausal symptoms
- Promotes the production of breast milk in nursing mothers

Celery

Apium graveolens

Celery is also sometimes called garden celery or wild celery. Either should work for these purposes. You're probably familiar with how celery looks when you buy it in the store: long, bright green stalks grown tightly together with delicate green leaves on top. If celery remains in the ground for a second year, it also develops small flowers that produce seeds.

The basics of celery

How many times have you munched on a celery stalk—without ever realizing you were actually eating a highly medicinal and beneficial herb! Just four stalks of celery per day has been found in studies to be enough to lower one's blood pressure.

In Asian and European folk medicine, celery has been used for hundreds of years to lower blood pressure, improve circulation, and eliminate or alleviate dizziness.

Celery acts as an all-around stimulant, which makes you feel more energetic. Celery also promotes sleep and has diuretic properties. All these effects may indirectly lead to an increase in sexual desire, especially in women.

Parts used

The root, stalk, seeds, and juice of the celery plant may be used.

Chemical content

Celery contains these substances:

- Apigenin, a muscle-relaxing substance that can dilate blood vessels and lower blood pressure
- Iron
- Vitamins A, B-complex, and C
- Phthalides, substances that act as sedatives and anticonvulsants

Dosing instructions and availability

Celery is available in several forms:

- Fresh, on the stalk
- Root
- Seeds
- Dried leaves
- Oil from celery seeds
- Extract made from celery seeds
- Juice

Fresh celery, seeds, and dried leaves are readily available at your supermarket. Oil and extract (made from the celery seed), and juice may be found in health food stores. You can even make your own juice with fresh celery. Use celery in recipes and for snacks. Tinctures or infusions made from seeds are usually taken ½ to 1 teaspoon 1 to 3 times per day.

What About "Frigidity"?

Even the word sounds bad: a "frigid" woman. It brings up all sorts of negative images. But it simply means a woman who has lost her sexual desire or libido. This can happen for a variety of reasons, whether psychological, medical, or both. But a woman doesn't have to live with frigidity. You can work with your doctor to find a way to regain your desire for sex. Some of these herbs may help.

Cautions

Don't use celery as more than a food during pregnancy because of its ability to stimulate the uterus and cause miscarriage. Some people also develop skin reactions when handling celery. Its diuretic properties could harm persons with kidney disease.

Added benefits

There are plenty of other benefits to eating celery:

- Lowers blood pressure and improves blood circulation
- May help control fat and glucose levels in the blood
- All-around feel-good tonic
- Acts as a diuretic
- Has a calming effect and works as a sedative, promoting sleep and more restful sleep
- Helps to alleviate arthritis and other inflammatory disorders
- Helps start menstrual flow
- Eliminates uric acid
- Acts as a uterine stimulant, may help to facilitate childbirth
- Helps with weight loss by promoting perspiration
- Helps the kidneys and liver function properly, which increases urine flow
- Used to assist the digestive process, contains fiber
- Helps to balance the body's chemicals, which may help with illnesses involving chemical imbalances

Chasteberry

Vitex agnus-castus

Chasteberry is a plant that is native to the Mediterranean. It is a deciduous shrub that grows from 6 to 18 feet high, and may also grow as wide as 15 feet. Chasteberry shrub is very aromatic, and has light purple-colored flowers that are followed by a reddish black berry.

The basics of chasteberry

Chasteberry has been used as a female hormone tonic in the Mediterranean region for thousands of years. An interesting thing about chasteberry is that it was actually used as an antiaphrodisiac, that is, to lower your sexual drive. However, it seems that it never did work well in that capacity. Perhaps that's how chasteberry got such a "nonsexy" name. Chasteberry increases sexual drive in women. It accomplishes this by normalizing the menstrual cycle and relieving PMS. It may even limit or prevent vaginal yeast infections. Some research indicates that chasteberry reduces prolactin levels. Prolactin is a hormone that occurs in high levels in women with menstrual problems. It is known that reducing prolactin levels resolves conditions such as amenorrhea. Other research shows that chasteberry relieves PMS symptoms. Relieving all these conditions may thereby increase a woman's sexual desire.

Some men report benefiting from chasteberry, too, but how this herb can increase sexual drive in men is unclear at this time.

Parts used

The seed or berry is used.

Chemical content

Researchers are still trying to identify the active substances in chasteberry.

Dosing instructions and availability

Chasteberry is available through health food stores or from mail order herb companies. It comes in pill, extract, or berry form. Follow labeling instructions carefully. The commonly recommended does is 20 mg of berries in tincture form taken daily.

Cautions

Chasteberry may affect other hormone therapies such as birth control pills, in vitro fertilization, hormone replacement therapy, or endocrine therapies. Pregnant women should not take chasteberry, since its effects on hormones are not well understood. A rash and stomach upset are the most common side effects of chasteberry.

Added benefits

Chasteberry is also used for the following:
- Eases female reproductive problems such as PMS and amenorrhea (lack of menstruation)
- Helps expel the placenta after childbirth
- Anti-inflammatory
- Increases milk production in nursing mothers
- Antifungal and antibacterial properties

Epimedium or Yin-yang

Epimedium grandiflorum, e. pinnatum, e. rubrum

Epimedium is a hard herb to find, but one that may provide helpful results if you are successful in locating it. The evergreen perennial has stems that grow underground, then grow upward, with leathery divided, heart-shaped leaves that change color with the seasons. Spikes of small, variously colored flowers appear in the spring.

The basics of epimedium

Called *yin-yang* in China, epimedium has the reputation of being able to give male hormones to women. In many parts of Asia, epimedium leaves are used in many food dishes.

Women may find their sexual desire increased when using epimedium. Perhaps this is due to testosterone-like substances that may be contained in the plant. However, information and research about this Chinese herb is limited at this time.

Parts used

Leaves are used to make a tea or are added to food dishes.

Chemical content

Active ingredients of epimedium and how they work are still unknown at this time.

Dosing instructions and availability

For tea, use 1–5 teaspoons of dried herb in 8 ounces of boiling water. Drink one cup per day. This herb may be available through health food stores. Also check Chinese herbal shops. You can also grow epimedium in mild climates.

Cautions

As with all herbs, pregnant women should use epimedium cautiously. Other information about cautions and side effects is unknown.

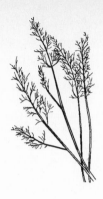

Fennel

Foeniculum vulgare

This hardy perennial herb grows in parts of Europe, the Mediterranean, and India. Fennel produces heads of yellow flowers on tall stems with feathery leaves.

The basics of fennel

Fennel has a rich and long history, including its use during medieval times, along with other herbs, to guard against evil forces, including witchcraft. The ancient Romans also used fennel for its aromatic fruits and succulent, edible shoots. Fennel also can satisfy hunger and once was used in medieval Europe by poorer people to stave off hunger pains.

Today fennel is used to increase the libido in both men and women. Fennel has been shown to increase the libido in animal studies using both male and female rats. Like anise, fennel contains an estrogen-like substance (estragole) and may thereby increase sexual drive in women. It was considered for use in the 1930s as a source of synthetic estrogen.

In men, fennel may interfere with testosterone, relieving bladder and prostate problems, thereby making sex more enjoyable. Fennel also moderates orgasm, allowing men to enjoy sex longer.

Parts used

The seeds (fruits), leaves, and roots of fennel are used.

Chemical content

Fennel contains the following substances:

- Estragole, an estrogen-like substance found in the essential oil
- Camphene cymene, a camphor-like solvent found in the essential oil and resin
- Choline, an amino acid essential to liver function
- Limonene, a lemon-colored substance found in the essential oil
- The minerals calcium and sulfur
- Oleic, petroselinic, and stigmasterol fatty acids
- Pinene, a substance similar to turpentine
- Vitamins A and C
- Other chemicals, including dipentene, fenchone, phellandrene, and 7-hydroxycoumarin

Dosing instructions and availability

You can find fennel seed and fresh fennel in most supermarkets. Other forms are usually available at health food stores. The seeds are usually what is used to increase sexual desire.

Fresh fennel can be steamed and served as a vegetable. For fennel seed, keep your daily usage down to 1 teaspoon per day or less. For tincture or extract, a common recommendation is to use ½ to 1 teaspoon up to 3 times per day. For seed capsules, use 2–3 455 mg capsules 3 times a day. For other forms of fennel, consult the product label.

Cautions

Using fennel as a food and fennel seeds is generally considered safe. However, do not use fennel during pregnancy—there is a chance it could cause a miscarriage. Fennel may be toxic if used in extremely large doses (1–5 ml), causing nausea, vomiting, and other problems. It may also affect liver function, so should not be used medicinally by anyone with liver problems.

Added benefits

Other uses of fennel include the following:

- Control PMS
- Relief of abdominal pain, gas, and flatulence
- Appetite suppressant
- Eyewash
- Relief of symptoms after chemotherapy or radiation treatments
- Flea and other insect repellent
- Relief of chronic coughs
- Promotes milk production in nursing mothers

Aphrodisiac Foods

Most of the herbs described in this book are used for culinary purposes. Experiment with creating romantic dinners incorporating several herbs. For instance, try pesto (which includes basil and garlic) over pasta, with steamed fennel, and cinnamon tea. The amounts of herbs contained in most meals won't reach medicinal levels, but perhaps even a little— or just the thought of sharing an aphrodisiac dinner—may lead to enjoyable sex!

Fenugreek

Trigonella foenum-graecum

Fenugreek is native to the Mediterranean, India, Africa, Egypt, Morocco, and England. It grows up to two feet in height, with leaves in groups of three. Small flowers produce the hard seeds that are used medicinally.

The basics of fenugreek

"Fenugreek" means Greek hay. A long time ago, it was fed to women belonging to a harem to increase their breast size, making them appear more desirable. Fenugreek has estrogen-like effects on the body, which may increase women's sex drive and pleasure. Research has shown that fenugreek does stimulate uterine contractions in animals.

Fenugreek may also relieve male impotence. Possibly, this may be due to the herb's ability to lower blood cholesterol levels, which may improve blood circulation throughout the body, especially to the genitals.

Parts used

The seeds of fenugreek are used.

Chemical content

Fenugreek contains these ingredients:
- Choline, an amino acid
- Diosgenin, a steroidal substance that increases appetite
- Essential oils

- Inositol, a type of alcohol
- The minerals iron and phosphorus
- Lecithin, a substance with antioxidant properties
- Mucilage, a gelatinous substance that help make fenugreek an effective poultice
- Trimethylanine, an amino acid
- Vitamins A, B (thiamine), B_2 (riboflavin), B, B_6 (pyridoxine), B_{12} , and D
- The chemical trigonelline

Dosing instructions and availability

This herb is usually available through health food stores as seeds or seed capsules. Generally, a 626 mg capsule is taken 2–3 times per day. Follow labeling instructions carefully. Externally, ground seeds mixed with water is used as a poultice.

Cautions

Pregnant women should limit use of fenugreek because of its ability to mimic estrogen and induce uterine contractions.

Added benefits

Other traditional uses of fenugreek include the following:
- Reduces fever
- Lubricates intestines and serves as a bulk laxative
- Helps eliminate mucus, which is good for asthma, sinus problems, and other lung disorders
- Aids in milk production of nursing mothers
- May help eliminate or minimize vaginal dryness
- Stimulates appetite
- Reduces blood cholesterol levels

Fo-ti or He Shou Wu

Polygonum multiflorum

This perennial evergreen vine is one of the main herbs used in Chinese medicine. It is also called knotweed.

The basics of fo-ti

Fo-ti supposedly got its Chinese name from a man who used the herb and became sexually active after impotence. Fo-ti is also used for a general stimulant and tonic, having anti-aging properties.

Fo-ti's general stimulant effects are said to also increase sexual desire and drive. When your body is functioning at peak levels, you're more likely to have higher sexual desire and drive as well. In addition, fo-ti's potential ability to lower cholesterol levels may increase blood flow throughout the body, especially to the genital areas. This would result in increased sexual drive and pleasure.

Parts used

The root of the fo-ti vine is used.

Chemical content

Fo-ti contains the following:

- Anthraquinone substances—emodine and rhein—that stimulate the bowels
- Lecithin, a fatty substance that may help lower cholesterol

Dosing instructions and availability

This herb can be found in herb shops or health food stores. It comes in powder, pill, or extract, and is also added to some beverages. Follow the label instructions on the product or contact an herbalist.

Cautions

Few side effects have been noted with fo-ti. However, limit its use so that your body does not become dependent on its laxative effects.

Added benefits

Other uses of fo-ti include the following:
- Diuretic
- Cholesterol reducer
- Aid to digestion
- Support of the endocrine system
- Anti-aging properties

Guarana

Paullinia cupana and p. sorbilis

Guarana (pronounced guar-an-A) is a climbing evergreen shrub with yellow-orange fruits. It is native to South America.

The basics of guarana

Folks in Brazil have long thought guarana to be an aphrodisiac. They make tea and even sodas out of guarana seeds, drinking it to get the herb's aphrodisiac effects. Guarana's powers of stimulation may make it helpful for stimulating the sex drive. It may also relieve PMS, possibly due to estrogen-like substances.

Parts used

Seeds of the guarana plant are ground into a paste that is then dried.

Chemical content

- Guaranine, which is similar to caffeine
- Tannins, which reduce intestinal inflammation
- Essential oils estragole and anethole

Dosing instructions and availability

Guarana comes as a dried herb or in pill, extract, syrup, or tea form. It may also be found in beverages. Check at health food stores or at markets that sell South American spices. Try 500–1000 mg of dried guarana or 0.5 to 4 grams of powdered guarana a day. Mix it into boiling water to make a tea, or add it to any soft drink. Follow labeling instructions.

Cautions

Guarana has the same effects as any caffeinated product, so use in moderation. Guarana colas may increase tooth decay.

Added benefits

- General stimulant and tonic
- Reduces fever
- Relieves headaches, including migraines

When Eating Seeds...

If you intend to eat seeds, make sure you purchase seeds marketed for that purpose. Seeds meant for planting have probably been treated to prevent rotting or disease, and such treatment may be harmful to your health if you eat the seeds directly.

Oats or Wild Oats

Avena sativa

Have you ever wondered where the phrase "sowing your wild oats" came from? The answer is right here from this herb: oats! Oats are annual grasses. You're probably most familiar with oats as oatmeal (ground grain) and oat bran (ground husks). Oats are also used when they are "green," that is, before the grain ripens.

The basics of oats

Years ago, stallions were fed wild oats, and it was generally believed that as a result they became friskier and had increased libido. Nowadays, men are hoping to become stallions themselves, while women may benefit in the bedroom from green oats as well. How green oats increase sexual drive is not really understood. So far, no studies have confirmed the ability of green oats to enhance sexual desire, though it has been shown to reduce desire to smoke. Perhaps, like other forms of oats, green oats lower the blood cholesterol, thereby increasing blood flow throughout the body, including to the genitals. Or perhaps they contain a substance that imitates sex hormones. Hopefully, further study will better determine how green oats affect the sex drive.

Parts used

The stem, leaf, and seed of unripe green oats are used medicinally.

Chemical content

Oats contain the following substances:

- Starch and gluten
- Albumin and other protein compounds
- Sugars
- Gum oil
- Salts

Dosing instructions and availability

If the primary purpose of your using oats is to enhance your sex life, you'll want to read the labels to make sure you are purchasing *green* oats. You can usually find green oats at health food stores or Chinese herb shops. Follow product labeling instructions for usage. A common recommended dose for tincture or drops is ½ to 1 dropperful 2–3 times per day.

Cautions

There are no known serious adverse effects associated with oats in all their forms.

Added benefits

Green oats are associated with other uses, as well:
- Antispasmodic, preventing or relieving convulsions or spasms
- Stimulant
- May aid in withdrawal from nicotine (the addictive substance in cigarettes)
- May make morphine medications more tolerable
- In addition, oat bran and meal can help lower cholesterol levels. Oat-based baths can soothe irritated skin.

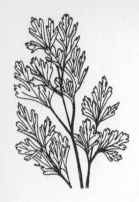

Parsley

Petroselinum crispum, p. sativum, p. hortense

Besides its use as a garnish for fancy meals or for cooking, the bright green, compact, leafy parsley plant can also be helpful to your sex drive. Chinese parsley (cilantro) is not related to this common parsley.

The basics of parsley

In folk history, parsley was used for many female problems. Women consumed it to increase milk production when nursing and to facilitate childbirth, as well as to increase their libido. Today, parsley is still used as a female libido builder. This may be due to its effects on hormone levels, which help regulate menstrual flow. Or parsley's high nutritional content may serve to increase energy, including energy for sex.

Parts used

Leaves and stems of parsley are used. For medicinal purposes, an oil is made from the seeds.

Chemical content

The following substances can be found in parsley:

- Apiin, a sticky, aromatic camphor
- Apiol and myristicin, which stimulate the uterus and reduce fever and are acids found in the essential oil
- The minerals calcium, iodine, iron, phosphorus, and potassium

- Mucilage, a plant gum
- Myristicene, a fatty acid
- Pinene, similar to turpentine
- Vitamins A, B-complex, and C
- Chlorophyll, a breath freshener
- Other chemicals, including bergapten, furanocumarin, isoimperatorin, and petroselinic acid

Dosing instructions and availability

Parsley is available fresh or dried at any supermarket. It is also easy to grow. Seeds or plants are available through most plant nurseries. Oil and root extract are available through health food stores. For medicinal purposes, place 1–2 teaspoons of dried leaves, root, or seeds in 1 cup of hot water (not boiling water—too much heat destroys the delicate oil).

Cautions

Large amounts of parsley oil could stimulate contractions in pregnant women. Long-term use of the oil can cause digestive irritation and other adverse reactions. Parsley oil can also worsen kidney problems.

Added benefits

Other uses of parsley include:
- Possible prevention of the spread of cancer cells
- Relief of gas, while stimulating the digestive system to function properly
- Freshening breath
- Diuretic
- Fever reduction

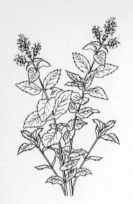

Peppermint

Mentha piperata

Peppermint is one of the oldest known household remedies and has been used throughout the world. It formerly grew wild in many areas, but now is highly cultivated to meet the increasing demand. Spikes of pink flowers top stems with oval-shaped leaves.

The basics of peppermint

In the Arab world, peppermint has long been used to treat impotence in men and increase libido. The American Indians used peppermint for a tonic and to help evacuate the bowels. Peppermint was chewed by the ancient Romans after eating large meals to soothe the stomach. This may be the reason why many restaurants offer peppermints after your meal—even though today's peppermint candy usually doesn't contain peppermint. The Greeks and Romans wore peppermint crowns at their feasts, and also used peppermint as a table decoration.

Peppermint acts as a relaxant to the lower muscles in the esophagus, aiding digestion while also eliminating gas, bloating, burping, and diarrhea. It also stimulates the flow of stomach digestive fluids. In addition, peppermint contains menthol, which cools and soothes the stomach.

The Chinese also have used peppermint for centuries as a medicine—it appears as far back as A.D. 659 in their medical literature.

Peppermint may aid sexual drive by increasing the respiration rate, which increases the amount of oxygen in the bloodstream. This in turn provides more oxygen to the genitals.

Parts used

Flowering tops and leaves of peppermint are used.

Chemical content

Peppermint contains:

- Essential oils
- Menthol, a type of alcohol found in mints that has cooling properties
- Methyl acetate, a fragrant solvent
- Tannic and other acids
- Vitamin C

Dosing instructions and availability

This herb is readily available dried and as a tea in most supermarkets and health food stores. You may also be able to find it fresh. Peppermint extract, tincture, or oil is available at some drugstores and most health food stores. Oil content varies considerably from product to product, so follow labeling instructions carefully. For dried peppermint, 1.5–3 grams is a common dose.

Use dried and fresh peppermint in teas and in cooking. Oils may be applied externally.

Cautions

Peppermint may cause a miscarriage, so if you are pregnant, don't use it medicinally. Menthol found in peppermint can be poisonous even in small amounts (1 teaspoon of menthol), so use peppermint oil cautiously. Peppermint may also interfere with the absorption of iron; therefore, if you choose to include peppermint in your herbal regimen, you should also increase your intake of iron-rich foods.

Side effects

Peppermint oil is recommended to use externally as a remedy for headaches. It should always be mixed with another substance, such as alcohol, since it may irritate the skin otherwise. Do not ingest peppermint oil, either, because it is toxic and only meant to be used externally.

Added benefits

Peppermint is used in other ways, as well:

- Increases energy levels and has anti-aging effects because of the increased oxygen in the bloodstream and better circulation
- Aids digestion and helps alleviate nausea and soothe the stomach (may be used after the first trimester of pregnancy)
- Contains antioxidants, which help prevent cancer
- Peppermint oil mixed with alcohol rubbed onto the temples is used to treat headaches
- Used to treat loss of appetite
- Used as a flavoring in products such as toothpaste and mouthwash

Quebracho

Aspidosperma quebracho-blanco

Quebracho is a tree native to South America.

The basics of quebracho

In South America, quebracho has long had the reputation of being an aphrodisiac for both men and women. Quebracho bark helps prevent the blockage of blood flow through the body and, as such, is considered to be an herb to help increase sexual desire.

Parts used

Bark from the quebracho plant is used.

Chemical content

The active substance contained in quebracho is a chemical equivalent to yohimbe, which is an herb whose derivatives are often used in prescription drugs to treat male impotence.

Dosing instructions and availability

Check health food stores and markets that sell herbs from South America. Carefully follow label instructions for dosage.

Cautions

The FDA keeps a list of herbs that it considers to be generally safe, and quebracho is on that list. However, it has been suggested that those with high blood pressure not try quebracho. The only reported side effect from quebracho users is dizziness.

Sarsaparilla
Smilax officinalis

Sarsaparilla is a prickly, climbing, perennial vine with long, creeping roots. Sometimes it is referred to as Chinese root. Sarsaparilla is native to the Caribbean.

The basics of sarsparilla

The most common American use of sarsparilla was as an ingredient of a soft drink similar to root beer. Medicinally, it was used by American Indian women as a tea drunk after childbirth to help expel the placenta. It is thought that the Crees used sarsaparilla in the treatment of syphilis.

Sarsaparilla has been used to treat frigidity in women, as well as impotence in men. It also has the benefits of raising the sexual drive in both sexes, perhaps due to the steroidal substances it contains.

Parts used

The rhizome (roots) of sarsaparilla is used.

Chemical content

Sarsaparilla contains these ingredients:
- The minerals copper, iron, manganese, sodium, sulfur, and zinc
- Essential oils
- Fatty acids, including sitosterol and stigmasterin
- Glycosides, derivatives of sugars

- Resin, an amber-colored sticky substance
- Saponins, sarsapogenin, and smilagenin, steroidal substances
- Sugars
- Vitamins A and D
- The chemical parillin

Dosing instructions and availability

This herb is available in some beverages found primarily at health food stores. You may also find it as an extract or tincture. A common dose is ¼–½ teaspoon of the tincture 1 to 3 times per day. Follow product label instructions.

Cautions

Sarsparilla is considered safe. However, doses greater than recommended amounts can cause stomach upset.

Added benefits

Other uses of this plant include the following:
- Increases energy
- Protects from radiation exposure
- Regulates hormone levels
- Acts as a diuretic
- Lowers blood pressure
- Helps clear up skin conditions, such as psoriasis, shingles, and eczema
- Acts as a laxative
- Relieves symptoms of inflammatory diseases such as arthritis

Saw Palmetto

Serenoa repens, s. serrulata, sabal serrulata

Saw palmetto is a small, shrubby palm tree native to the southeast region of the United States. It has sword-shaped leaves and produces dark berries about the size of olives.

The basics of saw palmetto

Saw palmetto has been used for centuries as a medicinal tonic, even by the Maya Indians, and it is thought to have been used even before them. John Lloyd, an American medicinal botanist, observed changes in animals that fed on saw palmetto. His observations included that they grew sleek and fat. This makes sense, since saw palmetto is known for being both an appetite stimulant and a natural steroid.

Saw palmetto has been used traditionally to increase the sexual drive of both men and women. However, it is unknown how the plant accomplishes this, as it contains substances that actually suppress testosterone. It is effective, however, in treating prostate problems, which can certainly interfere with sexual desire.

Parts used

The berries and seeds of the saw palmetto are used.

Chemical content

Saw palmetto contains capric, caprylic, caproic, oleic, lauric, and palmitic fatty acids as well as resin.

Dosing instructions and availability

You can purchase saw palmetto through health food stores and herbal mail order companies. It comes as pills, extract, and tea. Follow instructions on the label.

Cautions

Saw palmetto is generally considered safe. However, it can interfere with hormone therapies. Pregnant women should not use saw palmetto, as it can change hormone levels.

Added benefits

Saw palmetto is also helpful in the following areas:
- Relief of prostate problems
- Relief of urinary tract problems
- Anti-inflammatory problems
- Stimulation of the immune system

Yohimbe

Pausinystalia johimbe

The evergreen yohimbe tree is native to West Africa.

The basics of yohimbe

In the quest for better sex, the bark of the yohimbe tree has been one of the primary herbal substances used to increase libido and enhance sexual performance. While many herbs act as aphrodisiacs only on men or women, yohimbe has a long-standing reputation as an aphrodisiac for both sexes. In the past, people have tried smoking it and smelling it—now, though, yohimbe is generally ingested.

Yohimbe is often marketed as a "natural" alternative to anabolic steroids. Yohimbe is a precursor to testosterone, giving it a body-building capability. This makes it beneficial to those seeking to improve their athletic performance, along with their sexual performance. Another added benefit to using yohimbe is that many people find it lowers blood pressure. This could be bad news, however, if you already have low blood pressure.

Yohimbe works on improving the body's sexual functions by dilating the blood vessels of the skin and mucous membranes. This brings blood closer to the surface of the sex organs. Yohimbe also improves the blood flow throughout the whole body. For men, the result is quite obvious—bringing blood to the penis, allowing it to become erect, or more erect. In one study of yohimbe, where the participants were males suffering from impotence caused by psychological problems, 46 percent of the participants reported improvement in their erections and sexual performance after the herb.

In women, the effects are not quite so obvious, but most often result in a more pleasurable and intense sexual experience. This is how yohimbe has obtained its reputation as a libido and sexual performance enhancer.

Parts used

The bark of yohimbe is used.

Chemical content

There is one known active ingredient in yohimbe: yohimbine hydrochloride.

Dosing instructions and availability

The herb yohimbe usually comes in preformed tablets, capsules, drops, or extracts. It may also be found in teas and other beverages.

As with all herbal products, follow the label instructions carefully. Do not increase the dosage amount indicated on the label.

For prescription drugs that contain yohimbine, follow the instructions on the label, use caution, and watch for any unusual signs or symptoms.

Yohimbe should not be taken with foods that contain tyramine, which is an amino acid. These foods include cheese, liver, red wine, and some medications.

Cautions

Women who are pregnant or breastfeeding should not take yohimbe. Avoid yohimbe if you have low blood pressure. It may actually lower your blood pressure too much, resulting in fatigue and impotence. See your doctor first before trying yohimbe, especially if you have any of the following conditions:

- Kidney disease
- Irregular heart rhythm
- Psychological disorders, especially schizophrenia or manic depression

Side effects

Side effects associated with the use of yohimbe include:
- Change in heart rate
- Agitation, anxiety, or panic attacks
- Insomnia
- Hypotension (low blood pressure)
- Seizure
- Hallucination
- Headache
- Suicidal tendencies

Discontinue use immediately if you experience any of these symptoms and call your health care provider.

Drug interactions

Yohimbe has the possibility of causing a negative reaction when taken concurrently with mood-altering drugs, such as medications used to treat depression.

Added benefits

- Lowers blood pressure
- Relieves angina (chest discomfort caused by blockages in the coronary arteries)
- Boosts athletic ability

4

Increasing Your Sexual Pleasure

Setting the mood and desiring to have sex are certainly the first two steps to enjoying sex. But once the "game has begun," there are many ways to ensure maximum sexual pleasure. Herbs can help, usually by initiating a change in your body's chemical balance, such as increasing your body's production of testosterone, the "male" hormone that functions in *both* men and women to create your body's sexual response. Because of this chemical-changing role, most of these herbs are more effective when taken consistently over a period of time. Within a few weeks of taking the herb, you should gradually begin to notice a change in your sexual response, increasing your sexual pleasure.

Chickweed

Stellaria media

Chickweed is a small, weedy plant with round leaves and white flowers. While many people consider it a bothersome weed, chickweed is an herb that has been used for centuries by various cultures for a range of purposes.

The basics of chickweed

Primarily, chickweed has been used for salads and cooked greens. However, chickweed has external and internal medicinal uses too. The North America Chippewa and Iroquois Indians both used chickweed as an eyewash and also to treat wounds externally. According to folk remedy lore, chickweed is an excellent herb to promote weight loss.

Chickweed helps remove plaque buildup from the blood vessels, which increases and improves blood circulation. Its effect in improving circulation may explain its use for better sex, allowing for improved blood flow to the genital areas.

Parts used

The leaves of chickweed are used.

Chemical content

Chickweed contains these substances:
- Choline, an amino acid that aids liver function
- The minerals copper, phosphorus, potash, silicon, and sodium

- Inositol, a type of alcohol
- Vitamins B_6, B_{12}, C, and D
- The chemical rutin
- Steroidal substances

Dosing instructions and availability

Many people harvest chickweed from the wild. If you want to try this approach, be sure you find a reliable person or other source for identifying the plant. Also make sure it's not growing in an area that has been treated with herbicides or pesticides. Chickweed is often eaten raw in mixed green salads. Many people also like to steam it. Chickweed is also available in creams, tinctures, infusions, and capsules. A common dose is three 389 mg capsules three times per day.

Cautions

This herb is generally considered safe. Few side effects have been reported.

Added benefits

Chickweed is used externally as a salve or poultice on burns and boils. It may also be used internally on sores in the mouth. A bath in a tub of water containing chickweed is considered to be one of the most soothing baths possible.

Chickweed also reduces mucus buildup in the lungs, making it useful for bronchitis and in the treatment of colds.

Chickweed is also used, both internally and externally, to relieve breast pain and inflammation of nursing mothers. Chickweed is also a refrigerant, which enables it to reduce fever.

Damiana

Turnera diffusa

Damiana is a small, shrub-like plant native to Mexico. Although the plant itself is small, its popularity as a sex herb is huge—and growing.

The basics of damiana

The history behind damiana begins in Mexico. The story goes that it was an old Mexican folk remedy used to treat various urinary and sexual problems. Even the Maya Indians of Yucatan believed in the healing benefits of damiana. They called it *mizib-coc,* meaning "plant for asthma."

Generally speaking, damiana has long been thought to help a large and quite diverse group of ailments. From its being a laxative to being an aphrodisiac, you would be hard pressed to find a more useful herb available today.

Damiana has the reputation of being an aphrodisiac primarily for women, but can be helpful for men as well. A sexual rejuvenator, damiana helps when there has been a loss of vitality in the sexual organs. It does this by providing needed oxygen to the genital area.

Parts used

The leaves of the damiana shrub are the most commonly used part of the plant. However, it is not unheard of for some herbal preparations to also contain the stem of the shrub.

Chemical content

The damiana shrub contains the following:

- Essential oils
- Resin, a sticky, yellow substance .
- Starch
- Sugars
- Tannins
- The chemicals arbutin and damianian

Dosing instructions and availability

Damiana is widely available in health food stores. Many "mainstream" stores, such as discount stores and drugstores, now carry lines of herbal products, often even in generic forms. You may be able to locate damiana there. You can find it as pills, extract, or tea.

Even though there are no known side effects from taking damiana, it is generally suggested that you use it for two months, discontinuing usage if no positive effects are noted. Many herbs take at least four to six weeks to be of any benefit, so two months should be enough time to tell if it is helping you have better sex or not! Follow the dosing instructions found on the label. There is no set dosage amount, so if in doubt, start with a lesser amount, and increase if needed.

Cautions

While almost everyone would like to improve their sex life, a little caution is always a good thing. Damiana is not considered to be a very strong or potent herb, and there are really no known side effects. However, because there are also no scientific studies available on damiana, all we know about it comes from personal experience and its use in history.

There is some information that indicates that damiana may interfere with iron absorption. It would be a good idea, if you give damiana a try, to also increase your iron intake. This can be easily

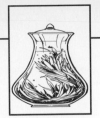

Drink Your Sex Herbs?

At least one company has taken an innovative approach to using sex herbs. South Beach (SoBe) Beverage Company has introduced a drink that includes among its many ingredients damiana, dong quai, fo-ti, and zinc. Langers Juice Company now has an energy-raising beverage that includes ginkgo and ginseng along with the juices of various berries. Of course, these and similar beverages contain very small amounts of herbs. However, you may want to try these types of beverages as an addition to a romantic meal!

accomplished by increasing the iron in your diet. Foods high in iron include dark green leafy vegetables, eggs, tomato juice, nuts, red meats, and fruits. You may also choose to take extra iron in supplement form. However, taking an iron supplement is generally *not* recommended for men, since too much iron in men is associated with heart problems. Ask your healthcare provider to check your iron levels if you have any questions.

Possible drug interactions

There is no current information on damiana's having a negative reaction with any other drugs or medications. However, there is some evidence that it may alter sugar levels in the bloodstream, so if you are diabetic or have any other type of problem with regulating your blood sugar levels, consult your healthcare provider before using damiana.

Added benefits

Just look at the wide range of physical ailments and conditions that damiana may help:

- Fights fatigue by acting as an energy tonic
- Relieves bronchial irritation and coughs, providing relief from respiratory conditions such as asthma, colds, and flu
- Improves and aids digestion and acts as a laxative by helping the muscular contractions of the intestines
- Helps regain strength in limbs
- Relieves irritation of urinary mucus membranes, providing relief from urinary conditions
- Increases fertility

Epimedium or Yin-yang

Epimedium grandiflorum, e. pinnatum, e. rubrum

Epimedium is a hard herb to find, but one that may provide helpful results if you are successful in locating it. The evergreen perennial has stems that grow underground, then grow upward, with leathery divided, heart-shaped leaves that change color with the seasons. Spikes of small, variously colored flowers appear in the spring.

The basics of epimedium

Called *yin-yang* in China, epimedium has the reputation of being able to give male hormones to women. After all, it's the male hormone, testosterone, that is responsible for the sex drive in both men *and* women. In many parts of Asia, epimedium leaves are used in many food dishes.

Men, in particular, may show improvement in the sexual function when using epimedium. Perhaps this is because of a testosterone-like substances that may be contained in the plant. However, information and research about this Chinese herb is limited at this time.

Parts used

The leaves of the plant are used to make a tea or are added to food dishes.

Chemical content

The active ingredients of epimedium and how they work are still unknown at this time.

Dosing instructions and availability

This herb is available dried in Chinese herb shops and some health food stores. You can also grow epimedium in mild climates.

Use 1–5 teaspoons of dried herb in 8 ounces of boiling water. Drink one cup per day.

Cautions

As with all herbs, pregnant women should use epimedium cautiously. Other information about cautions and side effects is unknown.

Fenugreek

Trigonella foenum-graecum

Fenugreek is native to the Mediterranean, India, Africa, Egypt, Morocco, and England. It grows up to two feet in height, with leaves in groups of three. Small flowers produce the hard seeds that are used medicinally.

The basics of fenugreek

"Fenugreek" means Greek hay. A long time ago, it was fed to women belonging to a harem to increase their breast size, making them appear more desirable. Although these claims have yet to be proven, research has shown that fenugreek does stimulate uterine contractions in animals. This is probably because fenugreek has estrogen-like effects on the body. Another benefit of the estrogen-like characteristics of fenugreek may be an increased sexual pleasure in women by eliminating or minimizing vaginal dryness.

Fenugreek may also relieve male impotence. Possibly, this is due to the herb's ability to lower blood cholesterol levels, which may improve blood circulation throughout the body, especially to the genitals.

Parts used

The seeds of fenugreek are used.

Chemical content

Fenugreek contains these ingredients:
- Choline, an amino acid that aids liver function

- Diosgenin, a steroidal substance that increases appetite
- Essential oils
- Inositol, a type of alcohol
- The minerals iron and phosphorus
- Lecithin
- Mucilage, a type of gum that helps make fenugreek an effective poultice
- Trimethylanine, an amino acid
- Vitamins A, B_1, B_2, B_3, B_6, B_{12}, and D
- The chemical trigonelline

Dosing instructions and availability

This herb is usually available through health food stores in the form of seeds or seed capsules. Generally, a 626 mg capsule is taken 2–3 times per day. Follow the labeling instructions carefully. Externally, ground seeds mixed with water is used as a poultice.

Cautions

Pregnant women should limit use of fenugreek because of its ability to mimic estrogen and induce uterine contractions.

Added benefits

Other traditional uses of fenugreek include the following:
- Reduces fever
- Lubricates intestines
- Bulk laxative
- Good for lung disorders
- Aids in milk production of nursing mothers
- Stimulates appetite
- Reduces blood cholesterol levels

Fo-ti or He Shou Wu

Polygonum multiflorum

This perennial evergreen vine is one of the main herbs used in Chinese medicine. It is also called knotweed.

The basics of fo-ti

Fo-ti supposedly got its Chinese name from a man who used the herb and became sexually active after being impotent. It is also used for a general stimulant and tonic, having anti-aging properties.

Fo-ti's general stimulant effects are said to also increase sexual pleasure. When your body is functioning at peak levels, you're more likely to have higher sexual desire and drive as well. In addition, fo-ti's potential ability to lower cholesterol levels may increase blood flow throughout the body, especially to the genital areas. This would result in increased sexual drive and pleasure.

Parts used

The root of the fo-ti vine is used.

Chemical content

Fo-ti contains the following substances:
- Anthraquinone substances—emodine and rhein—that stimulate the bowels
- Lecithin, a fatty substance that may help lower cholesterol

Dosing instructions and availability

This herb can be found in herb shops or health food stores. It comes in the form of powder, pill, or extract. It is also added to some beverages. Follow the label instructions on the product or contact an herbalist.

Cautions

Few side effects have been noted with fo-ti. However, limit its use so that your body does not become dependent on its laxative effects.

Added benefits

Other uses of fo-ti include the following:
- Diuretic
- Cholesterol reducer
- Aid to digestion
- Support of the endocrine system
- Anti-aging properties

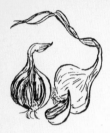

Garlic

Allium sativum

Onion-like stems bear purple blooms, while a large bulb made of many individual cloves forms underground on the garlic plant. Garlic is easy to grow simply by sticking individual cloves into the ground.

The basics of garlic

One of the most valuable herbs around since biblical times is garlic. During the construction of the pyramids in Egypt, the builders used garlic to keep up their endurance and strength. In more recent times, during World War II, garlic was used as an antibiotic to treat wounds, infections, and even gangrene. Garlic is even known as "Russian penicillin" because of its antibiotic qualities.

A Japanese study showed that garlic may slow physiological aging and age-related memory loss in test animals. One study done in Pennsylvania indicated that garlic may help babies nurse better. Garlic was given to nursing mothers one hour before nursing. It was found that the nursing babies attached to the breast better, nursed longer, and drank more milk.

Garlic's simplicity in no way detracts from its allure as a cure for everything ranging from the common cold to constipation. Garlic may be helpful for men in achieving and maintaining an erection by helping to dilate the blood vessels, allowing for increasing blood flow throughout the body. It may also help women enjoy sex more, by allowing for better blood flow to the body, including to the genitals.

Parts used

The garlic bulb and its cloves are used.

Chemical content

Garlic contains many helpful substances, including:

- Alliin, an amino acid derivative that converts to allecin, which has antibiotic effects on the body
- Methyl allyl trisulfides, which dilate the blood vessels, allowing for increasing blood flow throughout the body
- The minerals calcium, chromium, cobalt, copper, iodine, iron, magnesium, nitrogen, phosphorus, potassium, selenium, sodium, sulfur, and zinc
- Vitamins A, B_1, B_2, and C

Dosing instructions and availability

This herb is readily available in many forms. The produce section of your grocery store probably has fresh garlic bulbs and crushed, minced, and clove garlic in jars. Dried garlic can be found in the spice section. Garlic pills, including the odorless kind, are readily located in drugstores, health food stores, and mail order catalogs. You can easily grow garlic just by planting individual cloves.

Garlic can be added to foods while cooking, or garlic pills can be taken by mouth. Follow the product labeling for instructions. Common doses of garlic include 1–5 fresh cloves or 10–20 grams of garlic extract daily. French herbalist Maurice Messegue recommended that men use crushed garlic to massage the tailbone area in a circular motion for about 10 minutes a day to cure impotence.

Cautions

Besides strong breath and a garlic-like body odor, side effects from eating garlic are rare. They include nausea, vomiting, and diarrhea.

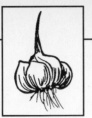

Try Roasted Garlic

For a delicious, sweet spread, try this:
Select a large garlic bulb and slice off
the top. Wrap in aluminum foil and bake at 350°F until
the cloves are soft (about an hour). Simply pop out a few
cloves and spread on warm French bread. The garlic is so
creamy and sweet, there's no need for butter.

Garlic may affect medications that lower blood sugar levels and thin the blood. Garlic can cause uterine contractions, so pregnant women should use this herb only as food.

Added benefits

The benefits of garlic seem to be endless—far too many to include in this book. Garlic aids blood flow and thins the blood by inhibiting platelet clustering, which reduces the risk of blood clots and heart attack and may prevent migraine headaches from occurring. Garlic is also known for lowering cholesterol, which helps to prevent heart attacks. It also helps in:

- Keeping blood pressure down
- Normalizing body fats
- Reducing the swelling of hemorrhoids
- Relieving fever blisters and herpes
- Soothing arthritis
- Aiding digestion
- Acting as an immune system stimulant
- Treating ulcers, athlete's foot and other fungal infections, bronchitis, candida, colds and flu, cystitis, and PMS

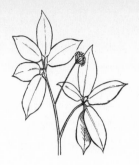

Ginseng
Panax ginseng, p. quinquefolius

A low-growing, shade-loving plant, ginseng produces red berries on stems surrounded by clusters of five leaves. The plant grows slowly, taking from two to five years for the root to be ready for harvest.

The basics of ginseng

Ginseng is an extremely expensive but wonderful herb that has been used medicinally for thousands of years. Its botanical name, *panax*, comes from a Greek word, *panacea*, which means "all healing." In China, it is sometimes referred to as the man's plant, referring to the shape of the ginseng root. Ginseng roots are considered to be more valuable because of their increased effectiveness as they age. The oldest roots available have been known to sell for as much as $20,000 per root! It is estimated that America, primarily the northwest United States and Canada, exports some $100 million worth of American ginseng every year; 90 percent of this ends up in China. Ginseng is sometimes referred to as the herbal "Fountain of Youth."

Despite its widespread use, no one is sure yet how ginseng works. Studies done by Russian scientists have shown that ginseng stimulates physical and mental activities and improves endocrine gland functions, while having a positive effect on the sex glands.

Ginseng may be a good herb to try for better sex. It has been known to fight impotence in men, by normalizing adrenal flow from the adrenal glands. This allows for an increase in the production of testosterone, a male sex hormone. Ginseng also is considered to possess healing qualities for the prostate gland, which may be inhibiting sexual function, too.

In some countries, ginseng is used to balance a woman's hormones during periods of intense physical changes. These changes would include the time after giving birth, during menstruation, or even menopause.

Women and men have reported greater sexual pleasure from the use of ginseng. This may be due to its energy-increasing properties as well as its effects on the endocrine glands.

Parts used

The root of the ginseng plant is used.

Chemical content

Ginseng contains ginsenosides, steroidal substances that affect the central nervous system and help the body adapt to environmental and mental stress.

Dosing instructions and availability

This herb is easily available in powder, pill, and extract form at your grocery store, health food store, drugstore, or herb shop. You can also find ginseng added to many other food products and beverages that are marketed as increasing energy. Common doses are 1–2 grams of root per day or 250 to 1000 mg of capsules. Amounts of ginseng vary considerably from product to product, so read labels and follow product instructions carefully.

Cautions

Since ginseng is overharvested and expensive, some unscrupulous manufacturers substitute ingredients. Purchase products that guarantee their contents, or buy ground ginseng root to avoid possible side effects from unknown substances.

Side effects from ginseng are rare, but include nervousness and diarrhea. Those suffering from hypoglycemia, diabetes, low or high blood pressure, or any heart disorder should closely monitor their symptoms when using ginseng. Also, women should not consume ginseng in large amounts, nor for too long, as it increases testosterone production, which is a male sex hormone, and may result in a lowering of the voice and increase of body or facial hair.

Added benefits

There is a long, long list of other benefits that you may gain from the use of ginseng. There have been reports of some athletes using ginseng to enhance their athletic performance, while also increasing their endurance. Many athletes also use it for over-all body strengthening and conditioning as well. Other benefits include:

- Fights fatigue, while acting as a stimulant
- Improves brain functions, such as memory, clarity, or alertness
- Helps heal the prostate gland
- Aids in the digestive process
- Reduces stress
- Regulates blood sugar
- Strengthens and stimulates the adrenal glands and reproductive organs
- Stimulates appetite
- May help treat infertility
- Increases mental alertness
- Helps to lower blood pressure
- Helps to prevent heart disease

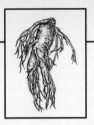

Three Kinds of Ginseng

Panax *ginseng from Asia and* panax quinquefolius *ginseng from America are both associated with increasing your energy for sexual activity. A third type of ginseng, Siberian ginseng* (eleutherococcus senticosus), *has medicinal uses, but may not be as effective in revving up your sex life.*

- Helps to condition the lungs, aiding in the treatment of emphysema, asthma, or chronic bronchitis
- Used to detoxify the body, aiding in the fight against addictions

5

Relieving Male Menopause, Prostate Problems, and Impotence

Men don't have such an obvious "change of life" as women do. But men face three problems unique to them that can impair their sex life: male menopause, prostate problems, and impotence. Male menopause and prostate problems strike many men at about the same time as women are entering menopause. Impotence can happen at any time, though it's more likely in older men. We'll briefly describe these three conditions and then list herbs that can help.

"Male Menopause"

We put the term in quotes because male menopause (also called andropause or viropause) isn't really the same thing as female menopause. Your reproductive system doesn't "shut down" and you don't lose the ability to father children. Furthermore, only about half of all men experience male menopause, whereas all women go through female menopause. However, in all men testosterone levels fall, starting at around age 40. If levels fall slightly and gradually, you may notice few, if any, changes. But if levels fall more dramatically, you may experience these symptoms of male menopause:

- Decreased sexual drive
- Impotence
- Depression, mood swings, and irritability
- Lethargy and insomnia
- Loss of bone mass

These symptoms are similar to those of female menopause. Also like female menopause, male menopause may be exacerbated by the major changes that are occurring in your life at this same time—children growing up and leaving home, retirement, financial concerns, or caring for elderly parents, for example. Other lifestyle issues can also make male menopause worse, including smoking, excessive use of alcohol, lack of exercise, and a high-fat diet.

If symptoms are severe, your doctor may prescribe testosterone replacement, medications such as Viagra, surgical procedures, or mechanical devices to aid impotence. However, all these treatments have serious side effects. Most men can benefit from quitting smoking (and all other tobacco use), reducing their use of alcohol, getting more exercise, and eating a low-fat diet. Herbs may also help, especially herbs that influence the body's ability to manufacture testosterone.

Prostate Problems

Many men commonly experience prostate problems as they pass age 40 or so, since the prostate at that time begins enlarging and tightens around the urinary tract (called benign prostatic hypertrophy or BPH). Prostate problems can affect your sex life in a variety of ways ranging from the inconvenience of having to stop activity to urinate to the serious complication of impotence. All prostate problems should be checked out with your doctor. In addition, many herbs may provide some relief.

Impotence

An occasional loss of erection can happen to any postpubescent male at any age and is usually caused by stress or fatigue (see Chapter 9 for more herbs that combat stress). But a consistent lack of erection—that is, impotence—is a serious concern. It's no longer assumed that impotence is simply "all in your head." Although impotence can sometimes be caused by psychological problems, usually there's a physical cause. Let's take a quick look at the causes of impotence. Then read on to see how herbs may help.

The causes of impotence can include lack of blood flow to the penis, nerve problems, hormone imbalances, use of drugs and alcohol, other health problems, and psychological problems. Some prescription medications used to treat these conditions can also cause impotence. Frequently, more than one cause is at the root of impotence, such as lack of blood flow to the penis and side effects from medication to regulate blood pressure.

Impotence Facts

- Impotence is more treatable than the common cold. Treatment can be successful in up to 80 percent of men with impotence.
- Half of all alcoholic men are impotent.
- About 25 percent of men over age 65 are impotent.
- Some 30 million American men suffer from impotence.
- Approximately 200 prescription medications may cause impotence, at least part of the time!

Lack of blood flow   Erections occur when you are sexually aroused and blood flows into the penis, making it longer and stiff. The penis usually remains stiff until ejaculation or orgasm. Anything that inhibits blood flow to the penis can affect your ability to have an erection. Heart problems, blockages in your blood vessels, diabetes, and smoking can all prevent enough blood from flowing into the penis. Getting treatment for any of these conditions and quitting smoking can help relieve impotence. In other cases, your doctor may recommend other therapies ranging from oral medications to injected medications to implantable pumps that create erections.

Nerve problems   Nerves carry the messages from the brain to your penis that signal the blood vessels in your penis to enlarge, creating an erection. Certain conditions can prevent nerves from relaying these messages. These problems include diabetes, muscular dystrophy, polio, multiple sclerosis, Parkinson's disease, Alzheimer's disease, and spinal cord damage. Controlling these conditions sometimes helps with impotence. Your doctor may recommend other therapies described above.

Hormone imbalances   A low level of male hormones, especially testosterone, can cause impotence. Testosterone levels fall in men beginning at around age 40, but usually do not fall to low enough levels to cause impotence. Abnormal thyroid function can also affect the hormones that are involved in controlling erections. Regulating hormones via medications can restore erections.

Medication side effects   Many common medications can cause impotence, including both over-the-counter and prescription medications. Blood pressure medication, diuretics (water pills), and antidepressant medications are all common causes of impotence. Usually medication can be adjusted or other medications can be tried.

Use of alcohol or drugs　You may think that alcohol helps put you in the mood for sex. But though alcohol lowers your inhibitions, drinking even small amounts of alcohol actually slows down your body's sexual response, making it take longer for erections to occur. If you combine drinking alcohol with another condition such as nerve problems, or if you drink an excessive amount of alcohol, impotence is likely to result. Street drugs can have many of the same effects on your sex life as alcohol. You may think you're sexier or you'll be more interested in sex after using such drugs, but the ability to perform when it counts can be greatly diminished. Eliminating use of alcohol and drugs is likely to help relieve impotence.

Other health problems　Cancer (testicular or prostate), infections, and sexually transmitted diseases (STDs) can all cause impotence. Cancer treatments such as chemotherapy can also cause this problem. For all these conditions, you need to work closely with a doctor to find ways to minimize the effects on your sexual performance and pleasure.

Psychological problems　Unrelieved stress, fatigue, and depression can all lead to impotence. Taking steps to resolve these problems can also relieve impotence.

When to Get Help

If you are frequently unable to have or maintain an erection, it's time to get some outside help. Start with your primary care doctor. Be honest about your problem. It's the only way your doctor can begin to assess the condition and find solutions. Ask for a referral to a urologist, a physician who specializes in the medical and surgical treatment of the genitourinary system. Usually urologists are the most highly trained, up-to-date medical practitioners when it comes to treating impotence.

Herbs That Can Help

These herbs may be beneficial whether you are dealing with "male menopause," prostate problems, or impotence. Also see Chapter 7 for information about health conditions such as diabetes that can cause impotence. And Chapter 8 describes herbs to help relieve stress and other factors that can make impotence more difficult to treat.

Ashwaganda
Withania somnifera

Ashwaganda is a evergreen shrub that grows anywhere between 2 and 6 feet in height. The ashwaganda plant has lush green leaves, small yellow flowers, and red berries. It is native to India, the Mediterranean, and Africa. Its name, however, may turn off some folks; when translated from its native Hindi, it means "smell of horse urine," which certainly doesn't make it sound very appetizing.

The basics of ashwaganda

Ashwaganda is just now gaining in popularity in our culture, and there is very little literature in English about it available at this time. However, for years it has been part of Ayurvedic medicine, which is the traditional medical treatment in India. Ashwaganda is thought to be India's answer to ginseng, another herb often used to increase libido. Ashwaganda is most often used to treat male impotence, but also has the reputation of helping to increase a man's fertility.

Part used

The root, berries, or leaves are used.

Chemical content

Known active substances in ashwaganda include the following:
- Ipuranol, an essential oil
- Withania, an alkaloid
- Withanolides, steroidal substances

Dosing instructions and availability

You may be able to find this herb in health food stores or herb shops. Or look for markets that sell Asian or Indian products. Ashwaganda root may be used fresh, cut up into pieces, eaten or brewed into a tea, or used dried. It is also available in capsule and powder forms. To make it into tea, simply add 5 teaspoons of the dried herb to 1–2 cups of boiling water. If you have some fresh ashwaganda and want to dry it, cut the root into small pieces and allow to dry for 7 to 10 days. Common doses include 150–300 mg of capsules (each capsule containing 2–5 mg withanolides) daily or 2–3 grams root powder 3 times per day.

Cautions

Ashwaganda is generally considered safe when used at recommended doses. Remember to take into account its sedative effects, however—especially while driving or operating machinery.

Added benefits

There are a number of other alternative uses for ashwaganda, including:

- As an anti-inflammatory
- For reducing stress
- As a sedative
- As a possible inhibitor of tumor growth
- As a possible antibacterial and antifungal agent

Barley

Hordeum distichon

Barley grows as a hollow-stemmed grass topped with long bristles that hold the rows of grain.

The basics of barley

Barley has been around for centuries; it was even one of the first crops planted in Virginia in 1611. Barley contains 11 times more calcium than cow's milk, and in years past was used to dilute cow's milk for infants. It is also one of the first cereals offered to babies. Plus, barley juice can be an inexpensive, natural way to help you quit smoking, which is a major cause of impotence. Barley also helps to reduce cholesterol while improving blood flow, fighting impotence, and reducing the effects of aging on the body.

Parts used

The green (unripe) grass and ripe grain are both used medicinally.

Chemical content

Besides a range of vitamins, barley also contains these active ingredients:

- Beta-glucan, a fiber with cholesterol-lowering benefits
- Chlorophyll
- The mineral calcium

Dosing instructions and availability

Barley is available in grocery stores as a grain, flour, or tea or in food products such as soups. Check health food stores for barley juice, tea, capsules, and powder. For appropriate dosages, consult the product instructions.

Cautions

Barley in all its forms is considered safe. The only known side effect is digestive discomfort in people who are unable to digest gluten.

Added benefits

- Lowers cholesterol
- May lower blood glucose levels
- Protects against colon cancer

Celery

Apium graveolens

Celery is also sometimes called garden celery or wild celery. You're probably familiar with how celery looks when you buy it in the store: long, bright green stalks grown tightly together with delicate green leaves on top. If celery remains in the ground for a second year, it also develops small flowers that produce seeds.

The basics of celery

How many times have you munched on a celery stalk without ever realizing you were actually eating a highly medicinal and beneficial herb? Just four stalks of celery per day has been found in studies to be enough to lower one's blood pressure.

In Asian and European folk medicine, celery has been used for hundreds of years to lower the blood pressure, to improve circulation, and also to eliminate or alleviate dizziness.

A study done at the University of Chicago confirmed that celery contains a compound that actually lowers blood pressure. Another study found that feeding rats the equivalent of four celery stalks every day lowered their blood pressure an average of 13 percent. Since celery improves blood flow and lowers blood pressure, it may restore erections in men whose impotence is caused by impaired blood flow.

Parts used

The root, stalk, seeds, and juice of the celery plant may be used.

Chemical content

Celery contains these substances:

- Apigenin, a chemical that relaxes the muscles that line blood vessels, allowing them to dilate and blood to pass through normally
- Butylidenephthalide, a chemical that helps start menstrual flow
- B-complex vitamins
- Iron
- Vitamins A and C

Dosing instructions and availability

Celery is available in several forms:

- Fresh, on the stalk
- Seeds
- Dried leaves
- Oil from celery seeds
- Extract made from celery seeds
- Juice
- Root

Fresh celery, seeds, and dried leaves are readily available at your supermarket. Oil, extract, and juice may be found in health food stores. You can even make your own juice with fresh celery. Tinctures or infusions made from seeds are usually taken ½ to 1 teaspoon 1 to 3 times per day.

Cautions

Don't use celery as more than a food during pregnancy because of its ability to stimulate the uterus and cause miscarriage. Some people also develop skin reactions when handling celery. Its diuretic properties could harm persons with kidney disease.

Added benefits

There are plenty of other benefits to eating celery:

- Acts as a diuretic
- Used as a general feel-good tonic
- Has a calming effect and works as a sedative, promoting sleep and more restful sleep
- When combined with coca and damiana, celery helps to alleviate rheumatism
- Eliminates uric acid
- Lowers blood pressure and improves blood circulation
- Acts as a uterine stimulant; may help to facilitate childbirth
- Helps with weight loss by promoting perspiration
- Helps the kidneys and liver function properly, which increases urine flow
- Used to assist the digestive process; contains fiber
- Helps to balance the body's chemicals, which may help with illnesses involving chemical imbalances

Damiana

Turnera diffusa

Damiana is a small, shrub-like plant with aromatic leaves, native to Mexico.

The basics of damiana

The history behind damiana begins in Mexico. The story goes that it was an old Mexican folk remedy used to treat various urinary and sexual problems. Even the Maya Indians of Yucatan believed in the healing benefits of damiana. They called it *mizib-coc*, meaning "plant for asthma."

Generally speaking, damiana has long been thought to help a large and quite diverse group of ailments. From its being a laxative to being an aphrodisiac, you would be hard pressed to find a more unique herb available today.

Damiana may help relieve the inflammation of the prostate gland, which is commonly a problem as men age.

Parts used

The leaves of the damiana shrub are the most commonly used part of the plant. However, it is not unheard of for some herbal preparations to also contain the stem of the shrub.

Chemical content

The damiana shrub contains the following:
- The chemicals arbutin and damianian
- Essential oils

- Resin, a sticky, yellow substance
- Starch
- Sugars
- Tannins

Dosing instructions and availability

Damiana is widely available in health food stores. Many "mainstream" stores, such as discount stores and drugstores, now carry lines of herbal products, often even in generic forms. You may be able to locate damiana there. You can find it as pills, extract, or tea.

Even though there are no known side effects from taking damiana, it is generally suggested that you use it for two months, discontinuing usage if no positive effects are noted. Many herbs take at least four to six weeks to be of any benefit, so two months should be enough time to tell if it is helping you have better sex or not! Follow the dosing instructions found on the label. There is no set dosage amount, so if in doubt, start with a lesser amount, and increase if needed.

Cautions

While almost everyone would like to improve their sex life, a little caution is always a good thing. Damiana is not considered to be a very strong or potent herb, and there are really no known side effects. However, because there are also no scientific studies available on damiana, all we know about it comes from personal experience and its use in history.

There is some information that indicates that damiana may interfere with iron absorption. It would be a good idea, if you give damiana a try, to also increase your iron intake. This can be easily accomplished by increasing the iron in your diet. Foods high in iron include: dark green leafy vegetables, eggs, tomato juice, nuts, red meats, and fruits. However, taking an iron supplement is generally *not* recommended for men, since too much iron in men is associated with heart problems. Ask your healthcare provider to check your iron levels if you have any questions.

Possible drug interactions

There is no current information on damiana's having a negative reaction with any other drugs or medications. However, there is some evidence that it may alter sugar levels in the bloodstream, so if you are diabetic or have any other type of problem with regulating your blood sugar levels, consult your healthcare provider before using damiana.

Added benefits

There's a wide range of physical ailments and conditions that damiana may help:

- Fights fatigue by acting as an energy tonic
- Relieves bronchial irritation, possibly providing relief from respiratory conditions such as asthma
- Relieves coughs due to respiratory conditions or even the common cold
- Improves and aids digestion and acts as a laxative by helping the muscular contractions of the intestines
- Helps regain strength in limbs
- Alleviates various cold and flu symptoms
- Relieves irritation of urinary mucus membranes, providing relief from urinary conditions
- Increases fertility

Damiana has the reputation of being an aphrodisiac primarily for women, but can be helpful for both men and women.

Ginger
Zingiber officinale

This perennial produces spikes bearing purple flowers, with knotty roots and rhizomes forming underground.

The basics of ginger

Although ginger originated in Southeast Asia, the Spaniards introduced and naturalized ginger in America. In fact, ginger eventually became so popular with Europeans, that in 1884, 5 million pounds of ginger root was imported to Great Britain.

Ginger is closely related to the herb cardamom. Besides having the ability to increase sperm count and motility, it also is said to help enable a man to obtain an erection. A study done in Saudi Arabia using animals, showed that feeding the male animals ginger, significantly raised the sperm count and the motility of their sperm.

Parts used

The roots and rhizomes of ginger are used medicinally.

Chemical content

Ginger contains the following long list of substances including acrid resin, bisabolene, bomeal and bomeol, camphene, choline, cineole, citral, gingerol (one of the main active ingredients, which prevents blood clotting), inositol, the minerals manganese and silicon, phellandrene, sequiterpene, B vitamins, zingerone, and zingiberene.

Dosing instructions and availability

Ginger root is available fresh, dried, powdered, candied, and pickled in grocery stores and health food stores. It is also available in health food stores and herb shops as an extract, tea, capsule, and tincture. Common dosages include 3–10 grams of fresh ginger per day, 2–4 grams of dried ginger per day, an inch square of candied ginger per day. For other forms, follow the product label.

Cautions

Using too much ginger may cause an stomach upset.

Added benefits

Some people report that using ginger reduces the intensity and severity of their migraine headaches. Some other possible benefits you may get from using ginger include:

Relief from both morning sickness and motion sickness, or any other form of nausea.

Relief from kidney pain; also promotes increased urine flow, allowing the kidneys to work more efficiently.

Ginger is considered to be an antiviral herb, which can help it combat many different conditions, including chronic fatigue syndrome and even sore throats.

Ginger helps soothes an upset stomach due to indigestion; it contains chemicals that soothe the stomach and it keeps the food moving through the intestinal tract.

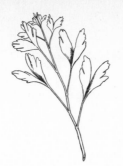

Ginkgo

Ginkgo biloba

This deciduous ornamental tree, native to China, has fan-shaped leaves and yellow seeds that give off a rather unpleasant odor.

The basics of ginkgo

Ginkgo is at times referred to as the "smart herb," because of its ability to enhance the memory and even possibly slow down the progression of Alzheimer's disease. Ginkgo doesn't perform miracles, but produces this effect by increasing the blood flow throughout the body, enabling the user to feel stronger and more alert. By stimulating and improving blood circulation throughout the body, ginkgo provides more oxygen to the brain, heart, and all other body parts, including those required for sex. This improved blood flow to the genitals may possibly help relieve conditions such as impotence.

One study conducted for a six-month period shows that 50 percent of the men regained erections when using ginkgo. In a nine-month study where the test subjects were men suffering from impotence due to atherosclerotic clogging of the penile artery, ginkgo gave 78 percent of the men improvement in their sexual functions. Add to this the fact that there were no reported side effects during this study from their use of ginkgo.

Parts used

The leaves and nuts of the ginkgo tree are used.

Chemical content

- Gingko extract contains the active ingredients of flavone glycosides and terpenes
- Gingkolides are steroidal substances in the tree, and are currently under research

Dosing instructions and availability

This herb is available in grocery, drug, and health food stores, as well as through herb shops and mail order companies. It comes in pills, extract, and added to products.

Follow the instructions on the product's label. It takes several months to begin to feel the effects of ginkgo. Many herbal practitioners believe that the amount of the active ingredients in ginkgo leaves are too diluted. To get enough ginkgo to be of much benefit, it is suggested that you take ginkgo in a standardized form, such as an extract or capsule. The usual dosing amount is 40 mg of extract 3 times per day or 60 to 240 mg capsules per day. Take this herb with meals to avoid stomach upset.

Cautions

Don't use more than 240 mg of ginkgo per day. Ginkgo can act as a blood thinner, so if you are already taking blood-thinning medication (including aspirin), avoid this herb. There have been reports of diarrhea, restlessness, and irritability when using ginkgo.

Added benefits

Take a look at what ginkgo may do for you:
- Lower blood pressure
- Help to prevent blood clots from forming, possibly preventing heart attack or stroke

- Improve mental ability, such as memory, clarity, and alertness
- May slow down the advancement of Alzheimer's disease
- Alleviate depression
- Provide relief from tinnitis, or ringing in the ears
- Relieve muscle aches and pains

Add to this list antiaging. By improving mental functions, helping blood circulation, and being an antioxidant, ginkgo may help you live a longer, healthier, fuller life.

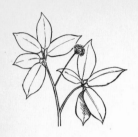

Ginseng

Panax ginseng, p. quinquefolius

A low-growing, shade-loving plant, ginseng produces red berries on stems surrounded by clusters of five leaves. The plant grows slowly, taking from two to five years for the root to be ready for harvest.

The basics of ginseng

Ginseng is an extremely expensive but wonderful herb that has been used medicinally for thousands of years. Its botanical name, *panax*, comes from a Greek word, *panacea*, which means "all healing." In China, it is sometimes referred to as the man's plant, referring to the shape of the ginseng root.

Ginseng roots are considered to be more valuable because of their increased effectiveness as they age. The oldest roots available have been known to sell for as much as $20,000 per root! It is estimated that America, primarily the northwest United States and Canada, exports some $100 million worth of American ginseng every year; 90 percent of this ends up in China. Ginseng is sometimes referred to as the herbal "Fountain of Youth."

Despite its widespread use, no one is sure yet how ginseng works. Studies done by Russian scientists have shown that ginseng stimulates physical and mental activities and improves endocrine gland functions, while having a positive effect on the sex glands. It has been known to fight impotence in men, by normalizing adrenal flow from the adrenal glands. This allows for an increase in the production of testosterone, a male sex hormone. Ginseng also is considered to possess healing qualities for the prostate gland, which may be inhibiting sexual function, too.

Parts used

The root of the ginseng plant is used.

Chemical content

Ginseng contains ginsenosides, steroidal substances that affect the central nervous system and help the body adapt to environmental and mental stress.

Dosing instructions and availability

This herb is easily available in powder, pill, and extract form at your grocery store, health food store, drugstore, or herb shop. You can also find ginseng added to many other food products and beverages that are marketed as increasing energy. Common doses are 1–2 grams of root per day or 250 to 1000 mg of capsules. Amounts of ginseng vary considerably from product to product, so read labels and follow product instructions carefully. (See page 84 for information on the different kinds of ginseng.)

Cautions

Since ginseng is overharvested and expensive, some unscrupulous manufacturers substitute ingredients. Purchase products that guarantee their contents, or buy ground ginseng root to avoid possible side effects from unknown substances.

Side effects from ginseng are rare, but include nervousness and diarrhea. Those suffering from hypoglycemia, diabetes, low or high blood pressure, or any heart disorder should closely monitor their symptoms when using ginseng.

Possible drug interactions

Ginseng may also interact with certain types of medications, both over-the-counter and prescription. More specifically, some antibiotic, tranquilizer, sedative, and antihistamine medications may interact with ginseng, so always use with caution and read all labels.

Added benefits

Women who don't have much desire for sex have also reported a greater desire when using ginseng. Some women have also reported greater sexual pleasure from the use of ginseng. In some countries, ginseng is used to balance a woman's hormones during periods of intense physical changes. These changes would include the time after giving birth, during menstruation, or even menopause.

There have been reports of athletes using ginseng to enhance their athletic performance, while also increasing their endurance. But there is a long list of other benefits that you may gain from the use of ginseng:

- Fights fatigue, while acting as a stimulant
- Improves brain functions, such as memory or alertness
- Aids in the digestive process
- Reduces stress
- Regulates blood sugar
- Strengthens and stimulates the adrenal glands and reproductive organs
- Stimulates appetite
- May help treat infertility
- Helps to lower blood pressure
- Helps to prevent heart disease
- Helps to condition the lungs, aiding in the treatment of emphysema, asthma, or chronic bronchitis
- Used to detoxify the body

Hydrangea

Hydrangea arborescens

A shrub growing to ten feet tall, hydrangea has woody stems with large, round leaves. Hydrangea produces clusters of white flowers. Note that this hydrangea is native to North America. It is not the same as those usually used as ornamentals. Nor is it the same hydrangea used in traditional Chinese medicine.

The basics of hydrangea

Its name was derived from a Greek word meaning "water-vessel." Hydrangea was once used by the Cherokee Indians as a diuretic and in the treatment of "calculi," that is, stones or deposits in the kidneys. It is still thought to be an excellent herb to purge the kidneys, as well as an overall tonic.

Hydrangea root may be helpful when prostate disorders such as infections and inflammation prevent enjoyment of sex.

Parts used

Only the roots of the hydrangea plant should be used.

Chemical content

Hydrangea contains these substances:
- Essential oils
- Saponin, a soapy substance
- Resin, a yellow, sticky substance

Dosing instructions and availability

This herb is available in pill and extract form from health food stores and herb shops. Follow the product label instructions.

Cautions

Do not use the leaves or buds of the hydrangea plant. They contain cyanide, and may be toxic. Over time, hydrangea root also may cause vertigo (dizziness) in some people.

Added benefits

Hydrangea has the following uses:

- Helps correct bedwetting in children
- Helps to evacuate gravelly deposits from the bladder
- Alleviates the pain from passing deposits from the bladder
- Acts as a diuretic
- Stimulates kidney function
- Helps treat obesity
- Acts as a laxative
- May be useful in treating allergies

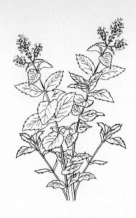

Peppermint
Mentha piperata

Peppermint is one of the oldest known household remedies and has been used throughout the world. It formerly grew wild in many areas, but now is highly cultivated to meet the increasing demand. Spikes of pink flowers top stems with oval-shaped leaves.

The basics of peppermint

In the Arab world, peppermint has long been used to treat impotence in men and increase libido. The American Indians used peppermint for a tonic and to evacuate the bowels. Peppermint was chewed by the ancient Romans after eating large meals to soothe the stomach. This may be the reason why many restaurants today offer peppermints after your meal even though most peppermint candy does not actually contain peppermint. The Greeks and Romans wore peppermint crowns at their feasts, and also used peppermint as a table decoration. Peppermint acts as a relaxant to the lower muscles in the esophagus, aiding digestion while also eliminating gas, bloating, burping, and diarrhea. It also stimulates the flow of stomach digestive fluids. Peppermint contains menthol, which cools and soothes the stomach.

The Chinese also have used peppermint for centuries as a medicine; it appears as far back as A.D. 659 in their medical literature.

Peppermint relieves impotence by increasing the respiration rate. This increases the amount of oxygen in the bloodstream, providing better blood circulation to vital areas, including the penis.

Parts used

Flowering tops and leaves of peppermint are used.

Chemical content

Peppermint contains:

- Essential oils
- Menthol, a type of alcohol found in mints
- Methyl acetate, a fragrant solvent
- Tannic and other acids
- Vitamin C

Dosing instructions and availability

This herb is readily available dried and as a tea in most supermarkets and health food stores. You may also be able to find it fresh. Peppermint extract, tincture, or oil is available at some drugstores and most health food stores. Oil content varies considerably from product to product, so follow labeling instructions carefully. For dried peppermint, 1.5–3 grams is a common dose.

Use dried and fresh peppermint in teas and in cooking. Oils may be applied externally.

Cautions

Menthol found in peppermint can be poisonous even in small amounts (1 teaspoon of menthol), so use peppermint oil cautiously. Peppermint may also interfere with the absorption of iron, so if you choose to include peppermint in your herbal regiment, you should also increase your intake of iron-rich foods. (Be aware that men should limit their use of iron supplements, since too much iron is associated with heart problems.)

Peppermint oil is recommended to use externally as a remedy for headaches. It should always be mixed with another substance, such as alcohol, since it may irritate the skin otherwise. Do not ingest peppermint oil, either, because it is toxic and only meant to be used externally.

Added benefits

Peppermint is used in other ways, as well:
- Increases energy levels and has antiaging effects because of the increased oxygen in the bloodstream and better circulation
- Aids digestion and helps alleviate nausea and soothe the stomach (may be used after the first trimester of pregnancy)
- Contains antioxidants, which help prevent cancer
- Peppermint oil mixed with alcohol and rubbed onto the temples is used to treat headaches
- Used to treat loss of appetite
- Used as a flavoring in products such as chewing gum, toothpaste, and mouthwash

Pygeum

Prunus africana

Pygeum (pronounced pie-GEE-um) is an evergreen tree with leathery leaves that grows in South Africa. It is related to other members of the *prunus* tree family, such as flowering cherry.

The basics of pygeum

Pygeum has potential benefits for men with prostate problems. However, pygeum is in danger of being overharvested, so it may be difficult to find in the marketplace.

It's a commonly used treatment for benign prostatic hypertrophy in many parts of Europe and in Africa. Certain substances in pygeum may reduce the swelling and inflammation of the prostate gland. Pygeum also has a diuretic effect on the body, which helps to alleviate another symptom of BPH, or frequent urination. Some men report relief of symptoms within days; for others, relief may not come for several months.

A study in Germany showed that pygeum reduced the swelling of the prostate gland. The study tested 250 men who suffered from BPH, with 66 percent of the participants reporting relief from their symptoms.

Parts used

Pygeum bark is used.

Chemical content

Pygeum contains plant-type steroids.

Dosing instructions and availability

You can find this herb in herb shops and health food stores, usually as a pill or extract.

Follow the instructions on the label. Many feel that pygeum works best when combined with saw palmetto, another herb that reduces the swelling of the prostate gland.

Cautions

Because of its diuretic properties, it is probably best to avoid this herb if you have kidney problems. Other cautions or side effects are not well understood at this time.

Added benefits

Pygeum is also used as:

- An anti-inflammatory
- A diuretic

Sarsaparilla
Smilax officinalis

Sarsaparilla is a prickly, climbing, perennial vine with long, creeping roots. Sometimes it is referred to as Chinese root. Sarsaparilla is native to the Caribbean.

The basics of sarsparilla

The most common American use of sarsparilla was as an ingredient in a soft drink similar to root beer. Medicinally, it was used by Native American women as a tea drunk after childbirth to help expel the placenta. It is thought that the Crees used sarsaparilla in the treatment of syphilis.

Sarsaparilla contains a testosterone-like substance that may be what causes it to increase sexual drive in men. Sarsaparilla's testosterone-like substances may help relieve impotence when low testosterone levels are the primary cause of impotence.

Parts used

The rhizome (roots) of sarsaparilla is used.

Chemical content

Sarsaparilla contains these ingredients:
- The minerals copper, iron, manganese, sodium, sulfur, and zinc
- Essential oils
- Fatty acids, including sitosterol and stigmasterin
- Glycosides, derivatives of sugars

- Resin, an amber-colored sticky substance
- Saponins, sarsapogenin, and smilagenin, steroidal substances
- Sugars
- Vitamins A and D
- The chemical parillin

Dosing instructions and availability

This herb is available in some beverages found primarily at health food stores. You may also find it as an extract or tincture. A common dose is ¼–½ teaspoon of the tincture 1 to 3 times per day. Follow the product label instructions.

Cautions

Sarsparilla is considered safe. However, doses greater than recommended amounts can cause stomach upset.

Added benefits

Other uses of this plant include the following:
- Increases energy
- Protects from radiation exposure
- Regulates hormone levels
- Acts as a diuretic
- Lowers blood pressure
- Helps clear up skin conditions, such as psoriasis, shingles, and eczema
- Acts as a laxative
- Relieves symptoms of inflammatory diseases such as arthritis

Saw Palmetto

Serenoa repens, s. serrulata, sabal serrulata

Saw palmetto is a small, shrubby palm tree native to the southeast region of the United States. It has sword-shaped leaves and produces dark berries about the size of olives.

The basics of saw palmetto

Currently one of the top-selling herbal products on the market today, saw palmetto is recommended by many "traditional" health-care professionals in the treatment of benign prostate enlargement. Saw palmetto has been used for centuries as a medicinal tonic, even by the Maya Indians, and it is thought to have been used even before them. John Lloyd, an American medicinal botanist, observed changes in animals that fed on saw palmetto. His observations included that they grew sleek and fat. This makes sense, since saw palmetto is known for being both an appetite stimulant and a natural steroid.

Saw palmetto can shrink the size of the prostate, alleviating inflammation and pain. This may have the result of eliminating impotence when prostate problems are the primary cause of impotence.

Parts used

The berries and seeds of the saw palmetto are used.

Chemical content

Saw palmetto contains capric, caprylic, caproic, oleic, lauric, and palmitic fatty acids as well as resin.

Dosing instructions and availability

Saw palmetto is available in pill, extract, and tea form at drugstores, health food stores, and mail order sources. Follow the labeling instructions on the product.

Cautions

Saw palmetto is generally considered safe. However, it can interfere with hormone therapies.

Added benefits

Saw palmetto aids in the following:
- Relief of urinary tract problems
- Anti-inflammatory problems
- Stimulation of the immune system

Wolfberry

Lycium chinese

This shrub produces berries and is native to China.

The basics of wolfberry

Wolfberry may be one of the "up and coming" herbs as more is learned about it. There is not much literature available to us regarding wolfberry and its use as a sex aid. The Chinese have used it for centuries, though, as an anti-aging drug.

A common cause of impotence, especially in older men, is a low level of testosterone. The level of testosterone in your body directly affects your ability to achieve and to maintain an erection. By raising testosterone levels, wolfberry may help reduce impotence.

In one study, men over the age of 59 consumed 2 ounces of wolfberry seeds every day for ten days. After the ten days, their testosterone levels were higher.

Parts used

Seeds or berries of the wolfberry plant are used.

Chemical content

Specific active substances in wolfberry are still being identified.

Dosing instructions and availability

This herb may be available in herb shops and some health food stores. Follow the instructions on the product label or consult an herbalist.

Cautions

Little information is available concerning cautions and side effects for wolfberry.

Added benefits

Wolfberry also has anti-aging properties.

Yohimbe

Pausinystalia johimbe

The evergreen yohimbe tree is native to West Africa.

The basics of yohimbe

In the quest for better sex, the bark of the yohimbe tree has been one of the primary herbal substances used to increase libido and enhance sexual performance. In the past, people have tried smoking it and smelling it now, though now it is generally ingested.

Yohimbe is often marketed as a natural alternative to anabolic steroids. Yohimbe is a precursor to testosterone, giving it a body-building capability. This makes it beneficial to those seeking to improve their athletic performance, along with their sexual performance. Another added benefit to using yohimbe is that many people find it lowers blood pressure. This could be bad news, however, if you already have low blood pressure.

Yohimbe works on improving the body's sexual functions by dilating the blood vessels of the skin and mucous membranes. This brings blood closer to the surface of the sex organs. Yohimbe also improves the blood flow throughout the whole body. For men, the result is quite obvious bringing blood to the penis, allowing it to become erect, or more erect.

In one study of yohimbe, where the participants were males suffering from impotence caused by psychological problems, 46 percent of the participants reported improvement in their erections and sexual performance after taking the herb.

Yohimbe also has the reputation of stimulating the production of testosterone. In fact, many of the most commonly prescribed prescription medications for the treatment of impotence or decreased sexual performance in men contain yohimbine, a derivative of yohimbe.

Parts used

Bark of the yohimbe tree is used.

Chemical content

There is one known active ingredient in yohimbe: yohimbine hydrochloride.

Dosing instructions and availability

Yohimbe is available at health food and drugstores. Medications containing yohimbine are also available by prescription from your doctor.

The herb yohimbe usually comes in preformed tablets, capsules, drops, or extracts. It may also be found in teas and other beverages. As with all herbal products, follow the label instructions carefully. Do not increase the dosage amount indicated on the label. For prescription drugs that contain yohimbine, follow the instructions on the label, use caution, and watch for any unusual signs or symptoms. Yohimbe should not be taken with foods that contain tyramine, which is an amino acid. These foods include cheese, liver, red wine, and some medications.

Cautions

Avoid yohimbe if you have low blood pressure. It may actually lower your blood pressure too much, resulting in fatigue and impotence.

Also, see your doctor first before trying yohimbe if you have any of the following conditions:
- Kidney disease
- Irregular heart rhythm
- Psychological disorders, especially schizophrenia or manic depression

Side effects

Side effects associated with the use of yohimbe include:
- Change in heart rate
- Agitation, anxiety, or panic attacks
- Insomnia
- Hypertension
- Seizure
- Hallucination
- Headache
- Suicidal tendencies

Discontinue use immediately if you experience any of these symptoms and call your healthcare provider.

Possible drug interactions

Yohimbe has the possibility of causing a negative reaction when taken concurrently with mood-altering drugs, such as medications used to treat depression.

Added benefits

Yohimbe is also known to:
- Lower blood pressure
- Relieve angina (chest discomfort caused by blockages in the coronary arteries)
- Boost athletic ability

6

Relieving Female Menopause and Premenstrual Syndrome

There are probably times in any woman's life when the idea of having sex is less than appealing. It may be due to feeling bloated and cranky before your period starts. Or perhaps sex is just plain painful because of vaginal dryness brought on by menopause. In either case, there is a lot you can do to make sex more enjoyable. First we'll describe the changes that happen during menopause and the symptoms of premenstrual syndrome (PMS) that put you out of the mood for sex. Then we'll list herbs that might help.

Female Menopause

The female reproductive system is truly complex, regulated by several hormones. Over time, these hormones decrease, causing the monthly cycle of egg release and menstruation to cease. Usually this process begins in earnest when you're in your mid to late 40s and is finished by about age 50 or so. This slowdown process is really called "perimenopause," while the resulting cessation of menstrual cycles is truly "menopause." However, we'll loosely call the entire process "menopause," since most of the herbs described in this chapter can be helpful for either perimenopause or menopause.

At first the changes may be so slight, you may not even notice that menopause has begun. Your periods may be heavier or lighter than usual, and gradually the time between them increases. You may begin to notice hot flashes or flushing. Lubrication of the vagina may diminish, making sex uncomfortable. You or those who are closest to you may notice mood swings. These psychological changes may result from the hormone changes themselves or from the stress caused by other events in your life at this time, such as having your children leave home or dealing with the death of loved ones.

Once periods have ended, you have entered menopause. During this phase, you may continue to have vaginal dryness, since you lack the hormones that would normally signal vaginal lubrication to occur. However, other symptoms such as hot flashes and mood swings should diminish.

Premenstrual Syndrome (PMS)

In many women the symptoms of PMS are minor. In others, the monthly cycle brings with it shifts in hormones that make you feel like you're going from Dr. Jekyll to Mrs. Hyde. Throughout the 28-day menstrual cycle, hormone levels change in an attempt to prepare your body for potential pregnancy. An egg is released by the ovaries, travels down the fallopian tubes, and then moves into the uterus. In the meanwhile, the uterus has been preparing for a fertilized egg by lining itself with blood and nutrients (the endometrium).

If the egg remains unfertilized, it passes through the uterus and out your cervix. The endometrium sheds, a process you know well as your monthly "periods." In some women, the endometrium builds up or spreads to areas outside the uterus, causing pain, a condition called endometriosis. Whether your PMS symptoms are relatively mild, such as irritation and bloating, or severe, such as depression and pain, herbs can probably help.

Herbs That Can Help

These herbs can help ease the symptoms of menopause and PMS. Read the descriptions carefully to see which would be best for your particular symptoms.

Alfalfa

Medicago sativa

This perennial bushy clover bears blue, purple, or yellow flowers.

The basics of alfalfa

Alfalfa was noted in 1597 by English herbalist John Gerard to be an herb capable of relieving an upset stomach. In the Arab world, they call alfalfa the "father of all herbs." It's no wonder, when you think of all the wonderful nutrients contained in alfalfa—eight essential amino acids, four times the amount of vitamin C as in a glass of citrus juice, and high levels of calcium. For women, this translates to relief from various "female" problems, namely menopausal and menstrual symptoms.

Hot flashes, mood swings, anxiety, night sweats—all of these may be relieved by alfalfa. Vaginal dryness and itchiness is also alleviated by the phytoestrogens found in alfalfa. Premenstrual symptoms of moodiness, anxiety, cramps, and anemia may be alleviated by alfalfa, enabling you to enjoy sex more. Alfalfa's reputation as a diuretic may be why it is also associated with relieving PMS symptoms such as bloating.

Parts used

Seeds, flowers, leaves, and sprouts of alfalfa are used.

Chemical content

Alfalfa is high in phytoestrogens, which act as estrogen in the body. In addition, alfalfa contains these substances:

- Alpha-carotene, a substance similar to vitamin A (beta-carotene)
- Amino acids
- The minerals calcium, copper, iron, magnesium, phosphorus, potassium, sulfur, and zinc
- Saponin glycosides (in leaves), which may help lower cholesterol and prevent arterial plaque buildup
- Vitamins A, B-complex, C, D, E, and K

Dosing instructions and availability

You can easily grow alfalfa sprouts from seeds. Seeds and sprouts are readily available at most grocery and health food stores. (Recently some sprouts sold commercially have been found to contain *e. coli* bacteria; if this is a problem in your area, carefully check the origin of your sprouts, or grow your own in a jar on the windowsill.) Alfalfa is also available in pill, dried leaves, infusion, powder, and tincture forms.

Add alfalfa sprouts to salads and sandwiches. For pills or other forms of alfalfa, follow the instructions on the product label. For dried leaves, use 1–2 teaspoons of dried leaves per cup of water. Drink 1–3 times per day.

Cautions

Contaminants have been found in some dried alfalfa products, so use a reputable source that guarantees contents. Alfalfa—especially the seeds—can cause systemic lupus erythematosus (SLE) to flare up in persons with this health condition.

Added benefits

Men who suffer from an enlarged prostate, and increased urination due to this condition, may also find relief with alfalfa. Alfalfa helps reduce the inflammation and swelling that occurs with this condition. Other benefits of alfalfa include:

- Relieves constipation by providing a healthy dose of fiber
- Relieves heartburn and indigestion by neutralizing acids
- Helps to prevent osteoporosis with its high calcium content
- Fights infections, including acne
- Purifies the blood
- May help prevent Alzheimer's disease by improving blood circulation to the brain
- The vitamin K contained in alfalfa is also thought to reduce morning sickness
- High in chlorophyll, which makes for less body odor
- Natural source of fluoride for strong bones and teeth
- Aids in weight loss
- Acts as a diuretic
- Prevents plaque buildup in the arteries
- Lowers cholesterol

It is also thought that alfalfa may increase the production of milk in nursing mothers, while also boosting the amount of vitamins contained in the milk.

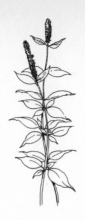

Anise and Star Anise

Pimpinella anisum

Anise is native to the Eastern Mediterranean areas, Eurasia, and Africa.
There are approximately 150 different
species of anise. All are notable for their feathery leaves and small
white or yellow flowers, as well as their licorice-like aroma and
taste.

The basics of anise

Anise is considered to be one of the oldest medicinal herbs. In biblical times, anise was actually one of the spices that folks used to
pay their taxes. The Romans also found good uses for anise, including eating a piece of anise-spiced cake to promote good digestion.
Anise helps alleviate menopausal symptoms, such as hot flashes. It
probably accomplishes this because of the active substance anethole,
which has been shown to exert estrogen-like effects.

Parts used

The fruit (seeds) of the anise plant are used for medicinal purposes.
Anise is readily available in the spice section of grocery stores.

Chemical content

Anise has been found to be high in anethole, which is a compound
with effects similar to estrogen, a female sex hormone.

Dosing instructions and availability

Anise seeds are readily available in the spice section of grocery stores. You may also find it as an ingredient in many food products.

The best way to use anise is to add it to recipes for baked goods and desserts. You can even find it in some herbal teas. The liqueur anisette also contains anise. Anise oil is also available. Follow the labeling instructions carefully.

Cautions

Anise is considered safe when used for food. Anise oil can cause vomiting and seizures, so limit use to less than a teaspoon per day. Pregnant women should limit anise to food use only, since its estrogenic effects could cause uterine contractions. Allergic reactions to anethole include redness and blistering with topical use or gastrointestinal distress when anise is eaten.

Added benefits

Other traditional uses of anise include the following:
- Stimulates milk production in nursing women
- May aid iron absorption
- Relieves painful flatulence
- Aids digestion
- Eases respiratory conditions, including asthma and sinusitis, by helping the body to clear mucus from airways
- Repels insects
- Promotes the production of breast milk in nursing mothers
- Increases libido

Anise is also widely used as a flavoring agent or spice. It is often found in commercially prepared cough medications and throat lozenges. It is also used as an antiseptic in some brands of mouthwash and toothpaste.

Black Cohosh or Sheng ma
Cimicifuga racemosa

Black cohosh grows native in parts of North America, most abundantly in the eastern woodlands. There are also some 15 species worldwide. This perennial is part of the buttercup family. It produces black roots and knotty rhizomes.

The basics of black cohosh

Black cohosh is commonly called black snakeroot, because of its traditional use as an antidote to a rattlesnake bite. In Chinese medicine, black cohosh is known as *sheng ma*. The American Indians have used black cohosh for generations for various gynecological problems, including inducing childbirth, inducing menstrual periods, and easing pain of childbirth.

Black cohosh reduces menopausal symptoms, including hot flashes, night sweats, heart palpitations, vaginal dryness, and vaginal thinness, by stimulating natural estrogen. Black cohosh balances hormones, strengthening the uterus and alleviating the pain of endometriosis.

One study observed the benefits of black cohosh in 110 menopausal women. Half of the study group received black cohosh. The other half was given a placebo. After eight weeks, blood tests showed significant estrogenic activity in the group of women who were taking the black cohosh. In another study of black cohosh, the participants were women with vaginal dryness caused by menopause. The results were virtually the same as the previous study—

the group taking black cohosh experienced a higher level of estrogen in their bloodstreams.

Parts used

The root (rhizome) of black cohosh is used.

Chemical content

Black cohosh contains these substances:
- Actaeine, a protein
- Estrogenic substances
- Isoferulic, oleic, and palmitic fatty acids
- The mineral phosphorus
- Pantothenic acid, a B-complex vitamin
- Tannins
- Triterpenes, substances similar to turpentine
- Vitamin A
- The chemicals cimicifugin and racemosin

Dosing instructions and availability

Black cohosh can be found in health food stores as powdered root or tincture. Some 40–200 mg per day of the powder is a commonly recommended dose. For tincture, a common dose is up to 1 teaspoon per day.

Cautions

Not much is known about the safety of black cohosh. Pregnant women and anyone using hormone therapy or birth control pills may want to avoid this herb since it can change hormone levels.

Added benefits

Other uses of black cohosh include the following:

- Astringent
- Diuretic
- Expectorant
- Relaxes and calms the nervous system, alleviating stress, anxiety, and panic attacks
- Lowers blood pressure and cholesterol
- Helps cardiovascular and circulatory disorders
- Relieves morning sickness
- Relieves arthritis
- Reduces the production of mucus

The Bad News About Black Cohosh

The supply of wild black cohosh is rapidly dwindling, because of its overharvesting. Careful cultivation of black cohosh will be required in the future to meet the demands of this popular herb.

Blue Cohosh
Caulophyllum thalictroides

Blue cohosh is an herb that grows 12–30 inches in height, with a spread of just over 1 foot. Native to North America, blue cohosh likes low, rich, moist soil in swamplands or close to running water. Like black cohosh, blue cohosh is gathered from the wild. It is feared that this plant, too, will become endangered before too long.

The basics of blue cohosh

Blue cohosh was used by the North American Indians primarily to relieve the symptoms of menstrual cramps, but also to help along childbirth, even to induce labor. The compound coulosaponin, which stimulates uterine contractions, is found in blue cohosh. Blue cohosh relieves menstrual cramps, especially back pain.

Parts used

The roots of blue cohosh are used.

Chemical content

Blue cohosh contains these ingredients:
- The minerals calcium, iron, magnesium, phosphorus, potassium, and silicon
- Coulosaponin, a soapy substance
- Gum
- Inositol, a type of alcohol
- Salts
- Starch

- B-complex vitamins and vitamin E
- The chemicals leontin and methylcystine

Dosing instructions and availability

This herb is available in pill and extract form through health food stores. Carefully follow the instructions on the product label or consult an herbalist.

Cautions

Since blue cohosh may help to facilitate and even to induce labor, it only makes sense *not* to use it during early pregnancy. Blue cohosh could cause miscarriage. It can also cause spasms of other muscles, such as the heart and intestines, which can be painful or even life-threatening. Eating leaves and seeds directly can cause stomach pain.

Added benefits

Other uses of blue cohosh include the following:
- Acts as a diuretic
- Acts as a uterine tonic
- Acts as a mild expectorant
- Helps to destroy or expel parasitic intestinal worms
- Produces or increases the production of perspiration, which may help in weight loss efforts or relief of edema
- Contains a steroid component, which helps to alleviate the symptoms of arthritis and common muscle aches
- May also alleviate the seizures of epilepsy
- Acts as an emmenagogue, which hastens menstrual flow

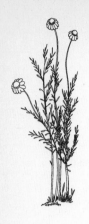

Chamomile

Chamaelum nobile, Matricaria recutita

This annual plant produces fragrant, daisy-like flowers. It is also called German chamomile, and is different than Roman or English chamomile.

The basics of chamomile

Chamomile tea and flowers have been valued for their healing power since early Egyptian times. Strewn on floors to freshen the air, used to cover up the smell and taste of rancid meat, and repelling insects are all early uses of this herb. As an antispasmodic, chamomile has been used for centuries to relieve the pain of menstrual cramps.

Parts used

The chamomile flower is used.

Chemical content

Chamomile contains these ingredients:
- Alpha-bisabolol, a substance that relaxes muscles and comes from the volatile oil of the chamomile flower
- Flavonoids, which have antispasmodic and anti-inflammatory action
- Chamazolene, an anti-inflammatory and anti-allergy substance.
- Polysaccharides, which stimulate the immune system

Dosing instructions and availability

Chamomile tea is available in grocery stores, drugstores, and health food stores. Other forms of chamomile, such as oil, are available from health food stores. The plant is easy to grow. You can collect the flowers, dry them, and make your own tea. Or purchase oil or tea at supermarkets or health food stores. Follow the instructions on the product label. For tea, use 2–3 teaspoons of dried flower per cup of water.

Cautions

Chamomile is generally considered safe. However, if you are allergic to ragweed or chrysanthemums, you may also have an allergic reaction to chamomile.

Added benefits

The many uses of chamomile can be summarized in three categories that cover a lot of individual ills:

- Anti-inflammatory
- Antispasmodic
- Anti-infective

Chasteberry

Vitex agnus-castus

Chasteberry is a plant that is native to the Mediterranean. It is a deciduous shrub that grows anywhere between 6 and 18 feet in height, and may also grow as wide as 15 feet. Chasteberry shrub is very aromatic, and has light purple colored flowers that are followed by a reddish black berry.

The basics of chasteberry

Chasteberry has been used as a hormone tonic in the Mediterranean region for thousands of years. It was actually used as an antiaphrodisiac, but never did work in that capacity. Chasteberry helps alleviate symptoms of menopause, allowing you to better enjoy sex. Chasteberry also helps alleviate premenstrual pain and dysmenorrhea and decreases fibrocystic breast tissue. It accomplishes these effects by causing the body to produce less of the female hormone prolactin.

Parts used

The seed or berry is used.

Chemical content

No one has yet determined the specific substances that make chasteberry effective.

Dosing instructions and availability

This herb is available in health food stores and herb shops as capsules, dried fruit, extract, and tincture. Follow the instructions on the product's label. Twenty mg of the fruit taken daily as a tincture is a common dose.

Cautions

Stomach upset is the most frequently reported side effect of chasteberry. It may also interfere with the action of other hormonal therapies and of dopamine receptor antagonist drugs, so this herb should not be taken if you are using any of these treatments.

Added benefits

- Antibacterial effects
- Anti-inflammatory properties
- Antifungal properties

Damiana

Turnera diffusa

Damiana is a small, shrub-like plant native to Mexico.

The basics of damiana

The history behind damiana begins in Mexico. The story goes that it was an old Mexican folk remedy used to treat various urinary and sexual problems. Even the Maya Indians of Yucatan believed in the healing benefits of damiana. They called it *mizib-coc,* meaning "plant for asthma."

Damiana may help alleviate the symptoms of menopause, primarily the hot flashes associated with it. It may shorten the duration of hot flashes while also decreasing the intensity of them. Exactly how it works in the body is yet unknown.

Parts used

The leaves of the damiana shrub are the most commonly used part of the plant. However, it is not unheard of for some herbal preparations to also contain the stem of the shrub.

Chemical content

The damiana shrub contains the following:
- The chemicals arbutin and damianian
- Essential oils
- Resin, a sticky, yellow substance
- Starch
- Sugars
- Tannins

Dosing instructions and availability

Damiana is widely available in health food stores. Many "mainstream" stores, such as discount stores and drugstores, now carry lines of herbal products, often even in generic forms. You may be able to locate damiana there. You can find it as pills or extract or tea.

Even though there are no known side effects from taking damiana, it is generally suggested that you use it for two months, discontinuing usage if no positive effects are noted. Many herbs take at least four to six weeks to be of any benefit, so two months should be enough time to tell if it is helping you have better sex or not! Follow the dosing instructions found on the label. There is no set dosage amount, so if in doubt, start with a lesser amount, and increase if needed.

Cautions

While almost everyone would like to improve their sex life, a little caution is always a good thing. Damiana is not considered to be a very strong or potent herb, and there are really no known side effects. However, because there are also no scientific studies available on damiana, all we know about it comes from personal experience and its use in history.

There is some information that indicates that damiana may interfere with iron absorption. Therefore, it would be a good idea, if you give damiana a try, to also increase your iron intake. This can be easily accomplished by increasing the iron in your diet. Foods high in iron include: dark green leafy vegetables, eggs, tomato juice, nuts, red meats, and fruits. You may also choose to take extra iron in supplement form. Ask your healthcare provider to check your iron levels if you have any questions.

Possible drug interactions

There is no current information on damiana's having a negative reaction with any other drugs or medications. However, there is some evidence that it may alter sugar levels in the bloodstream, so if you are diabetic or have any other type of problem with regulating your blood sugar levels, consult your healthcare provider before using damiana.

Added benefits

There are a wide range of physical ailments and conditions that damiana may help:

- Fights fatigue by acting as an energy tonic
- Relieves bronchial irritation, possibly providing relief from respiratory conditions such as asthma
- Relieves coughs due to respiratory conditions or even the common cold
- Improves and aids digestion and acts as a laxative by helping the muscular contractions of the intestines
- Helps regain strength in limbs
- Alleviates various cold and flu symptoms
- Relieves irritation of urinary mucus membranes, providing relief from urinary conditions
- Increases fertility

Dong Quai

Angelica sinensis

This perennial has purple stems, clusters of white flowers, and thick, branched roots.

The basics of dong quai

Dong quai is often called the woman's herb because of its tremendous reputation for alleviating various female symptoms. Records as far back as 588 B.C. show dong quai recommended for the treatment of painful menstrual cycles. In both China and Japan, dong quai has long held a reputation as "women's ginseng" and is second in sales only to licorice root. Its Latin name, *Angelica,* comes from the legend that its healing powers were revealed in a dream. An angel supposedly told the dreamer that it was a cure for the plague. Dong quai also used to be known as the "root of the Holy Ghost."

Dong quai balances female hormones, alleviating the pain and frustration of menstrual cycles and menopause. Some women report an increase in breast size after using dong quai. Used after childbirth, dong quai is considered to be a good postpartum tonic.

Hot flashes, anxiety, and mood swings all may be relieved by using dong quai, allowing you to enjoy sex more. Dong quai can moisturize the vaginal area and provide relief from vaginal dryness and itchiness, making intercourse more pleasant.

Parts used

Dong quai roots are used.

Chemical content

Dong quai contains several known ingredients, some of which can be harmful when used in purified forms. Ingredients include the following:

- Phytoestrogens, which act like estrogen in a woman's body
- Psoralen, bergapten, and other coumarin derivatives, which dilate blood vessels and relax muscles
- Safrole, a substance found in the essential oil, which in pure form can cause cancer

Dosing instructions and availability

This herb is available in herb shops and health food stores. Dong quai comes as a capsule, extract, powder, and other forms. It is also included in some beverages marketed to enhance sexual pleasure. Often, it is an ingredient in Chinese soups. When taking the capsule, extract, powder, or other medicinal forms, follow instructions on the product's label. A common dose is 3–5 grams per day. Avoid purified forms of dong quai because purified safrole can cause cancer.

Cautions

Dong quai can cause miscarriage. Coumarin derivatives may cause sun sensitivity and cancer.

Added benefits

Even though dong quai is best known for its female healing properties, it also has many other benefits. Dong quai contains compounds that are similar to prescription medications used to treat high blood pressure. For this reason, dong quai may be helpful for those suffering from high blood pressure or even angina or other heart diseases. Besides acting like a sedative for men, it is sometimes used to prevent testicular diseases.

Dong quai also has antibiotic qualities, quite possibly being able to keep you from getting sick. It is a blood builder, which helps to heal all wounds and treat those who suffer from anemia. It is a bowel lubricant, helping those who suffer from constipation.

Other benefits of dong quai include the following:

- Enhances vitamin E activity in those who are deficient
- Relieves insomnia
- Nourishes the brain
- Relieves arthritis pain
- Acts as an expectorant to treat bronchial conditions or coughs
- Helps to relieve gas and indigestion
- By increasing estrogen levels, dong quai may be used in the treatment of infertility
- May stimulate the appetite

False Unicorn Root

Chamaelirium luteum

This member of the lily family is native to North America. It has a base of leaves, a tall stem, and a spike of white flowers, which turn to yellow. It is also called helonias.

The basics of false unicorn root

Originally used as a Native American cure for conditions ranging from digestive problems to pain, false unicorn root is often recommended by modern-day midwives to their expectant patients, to prevent miscarriage. It also helps alleviate morning sickness during the first trimester of pregnancy.

False unicorn root's ability to balance the sex hormones in your body makes it useful for a number of "female" problems. This herb's reputation may be a result of its steroidal substances, which influence hormones, though how it actually works has not yet been determined. Women who are in their menopausal years or who have had a hysterectomy may find relief of symptoms such as hot flashes and mood swings. False unicorn root also may be used to help regulate a woman's periods, especially for those who have used contraceptives long-term. Women who suffer through the monthly woes of premenstrual syndrome or even endometriosis also may find relief of pain. Some women have even reported that using false unicorn on a regular basis helped them overcome infertility.

Parts used

Roots and rhizomes of false unicorn are used.

Chemical content

False unicorn contains chamaelirin, a strong antiseptic and steroid. It also contains numerous fatty acids and other steroid-like substances.

Dosing instructions and availability

False unicorn is available as an infusion, extract, or tincture through health food stores. It is also found in herb blends. A common dose is 2–4 ml of the extract taken daily.

Cautions

Not much is known about the safety of false unicorn. It may cause nausea and vomiting.

Added benefits

Men who suffer from an enlarged prostate and/or impotence may find relief by using false unicorn root, as it may help reduce the swelling of the prostate gland. Other benefits of using false unicorn root include:

- Diuretic action
- Ability to rid the body of worms and other parasites

Feverfew

Tanacetum parthenium

Feverfew, a perennial plant, grows wild in North America and other places throughout the world as a two-foot tall, hedge-like plant with yellow daisy-like flowers. This herb is also called featherfew and featherfoil.

The basics of feverfew

The word *feverfew* comes from the Latin word *febrifugia*, which translates to "driver-out of fevers." Since the Middle Ages, this herb has been used for just that purpose. Currently, though, feverfew has been making quite a name for itself as a result of its success in treating headaches—not just any old headache, but migraine headaches.

Feverfew has also been known to promote menstruation and to alleviate menstrual cramps. It also may help with the symptoms of menopause. It is thought that the same substances in feverfew that help relieve migraine pain also act to relieve these more "female" symptoms.

Parts used

Bark, dried flowers, and leaves of feverfew are used.

Chemical content

- Bomeol
- Camphor
- Parthenolide, the primary substance believed responsible for pain relief

- Pyrethrins
- Santamarin
- Sesqueterpine lactones, chemicals that may have both anti-pain and antispasmodic properties

Dosing instructions and availability

Feverfew may be made into a tea, though most will find it better to take feverfew in capsule or extract form. Feverfew leaves are known to have an unpleasant taste, and may cause mouth sores and inflammation of the tongue and mouth. It is generally recommended that you take between 60 and 380 mg of the capsules, or 4–8 ml of extract, per day; however, concentrations of parthenolide vary from product to product, so follow the label instructions carefully.

Cautions

Feverfew is generally considered safe. The most common side effect is mouth ulcers. Pregnant women should never use feverfew. Because of its ability to cause uterine contractions, it could also possibly cause a miscarriage. It is also suggested that nursing mothers do not use feverfew, either. Feverfew may also affect drugs used to prevent clots, such as aspirin, heparin, and warfarin.

Added benefits

By taking feverfew on a regular basis, many migraine sufferers have experienced a reduction in the number and severity of headaches. To find this relief, however, feverfew must be taken on a daily basis. It works as a preventative, and shouldn't just be taken when sufferers feel a migraine headache coming on.

Feverfew works to prevent migraines by inhibiting the production of prostaglandins, substances that are known to constrict and dilate blood vessels to the brain and may cause migraine headaches. One study shows that two-thirds of those who suffer from migraine headaches and were given feverfew were able to prevent migraine headaches.

Although best known for its headache relief, feverfew is often used as an all-around pain reliever. Here are some other benefits of using feverfew:

- Relief from allergies
- Relief of muscle pain and tension
- Stimulation of appetite
- Stimulation of uterine contractions
- Control of nausea

Flax

Linum usitatissimum

Flax, also known as linseed, has thin stems topped with branches of small blue flowers. This herb grows all over the world.

The basics of flax

Flax has been used by various cultures for years. It has even been found in various forms—such as seeds and cloth—in Egyptian tombs. Flax is cultivated in so many locations that its origin can not be established. This herb has properties similar to fenugreek, with similar effects on the body as well.

For many years, various cultures have used flax seed in the treatment of female disorders. It was described years ago as a remedy for "pains of the breast." Recent studies have shown flax to alter female hormone levels, which may help relieve PMS and menopausal symptoms.

Parts used

Seeds and oil from seeds of flax are used.

Chemical content

- Beta-carotene, the precursor to vitamin A
- Glycosides, types of steroidal substances
- Gum
- Linamarin
- Linoleic and oleic acids, the essential fatty acid oils thought to have many health benefits similar to oils found in fish

- Mucilage, a glutinous fiber
- Protein
- Saturated acids
- Tannins
- Wax
- Vitamin E

Dosing instructions and availability

Flax is available as capsule, oil, poultice, and seeds through health food stores. Common doses are 1 tablespoon of whole or crushed seeds 2–3 times per day or one 1,300 mg capsule taken daily.

Cautions

Because of its high oil content, flax is considerably higher in calories than many other herbs, so account for these calories by cutting out other foods. There are few known side effects from flax. There have been reports of people having toxic reactions to flax that contained small amounts of poisonous substances. You can probably avoid this potential problem by making sure that the flax you purchase is intended to be used by humans.

Added benefits

Flax may be used for many other ailments and conditions, including the following:

- To prevent constipation (Flax contains a lot of bulk and is an excellent source of fiber. However, remember to increase your intake of water to keep the bulk moving through your system properly.)
- A natural diuretic
- Flaxseed tea coats the digestive tract, protecting the body from ulcer irritations

- Relief of psoriasis (Flax oil is chemically similar to fish oil, which is known to relieve psoriasis and promote healthy skin.)
- To strengthen and regulate immune system functions
- To promote stronger teeth, nails, and bones
- Helps to relieve inflammation
- Helps protect the heart because of its high content of alpha-linolenic acid

Ginger

Zingiber officinale

This perennial produces spikes bearing purple flowers, with knotty roots and rhizomes forming underground.

The basics of ginger

Although ginger originated in Southeast Asia, the Spaniards introduced and naturalized ginger in America. In fact, ginger eventually became so popular with Europeans, that in 1884, 5 million pounds of ginger root was imported to Great Britain.

Sometimes women, as well as men, just aren't in the "mood" for sex. In some countries, in the local marketplaces, you'll find merchants selling ginger to "warm" up "cold" women. There may not be any scientific research to back up their claims, but ginger is tasty and and harmless enough so there's no reason not to give it a try!

Ginger is used by many women around the world to both relieve the pain and cramps of their menstrual periods, and regulate periods and their blood flow. It is thought that ginger contains six different compounds that relieve pain as well as containing six anti-cramping compounds.

Parts used

The roots and rhizomes of ginger are used medicinally.

Chemical content

Ginger contains the following long list of substances including acrid resin, bisabolene, bomeal and bomeol, camphene, choline, cineole, citral, gingerol (one of the main active ingredients, which prevents blood clotting), inositol, the minerals manganese and silicon, phellandrene, sequiterpene, B vitamins, zingerone, and zingiberene.

Dosing instructions and availability

Ginger root is available fresh, dried, powdered, candied, and pickled in grocery stores and health food stores. It is also available in health food stores and herb shops as an extract, tea, capsule, and tincture. Common dosages include 3–10 grams of fresh ginger per day, 2–4 grams of dried ginger per day, an inch square of candied ginger per day. For other forms, follow the product label.

Cautions

Using too much ginger may cause an stomach upset.

Added benefits

Those folks who suffer from migraine headaches are always looking for a better cure. Some people report that using ginger reduces the intensity and severity of their migraine headaches. Some other possible benefits you may get from using ginger include:

Relief from both morning sickness and motion sickness, or any other form of nausea—try one cup of ginger tea first thing in the morning or before driving/riding in a car, boat or other vehicle.

Relief from kidney pain; also promotes increased urine flow, allowing the kidneys to work more efficiently. Press hot compresses soaked in ginger tea to your lower back to alleviate kidney pain.

Ginger is considered to be an antiviral herb, which can help it combat many different conditions, including chronic fatigue syndrome and even sore throats.

Ginger helps soothes an upset stomach due to indigestion; it contains chemicals that soothe the stomach and it keeps the food moving through the intestinal tract.

Goldenseal

Hydrastis canadensis

A moisture-loving perennial, goldenseal has tall, straight stems with large leaves, whitish-green flowers, orange berries, and yellow, knotty rhizomes. It grows in wooded areas on the East Coast of North America.

The basics of goldenseal

Goldenseal is best known for its ability to act as a natural antibiotic. Lesser known is its ability to regulate periods, decrease vaginal bleeding, and treat vaginal infections. Hydrastine, a substance found in goldenseal, constricts blood vessels and promotes blood clotting, which may stop or slow down excessive uterine bleeding. Berberine, an antibacterial substance contained in goldenseal, makes this herb useful as a vaginal douche, allowing it to fight infection while also alleviating unwanted vaginal itching. It may also serve as an antispasmodic, relieving menstrual cramps.

Parts used

Roots and rhizomes of goldenseal are used.

Chemical content

Goldenseal contains the following substances:

- Albumin
- B-complex vitamins
- Berberine and hydrastine, antibacterial substances with anti-tumor properties

- Candine
- Chlorine
- Choline, an amino acid
- Chologenic acid
- Essential oils
- Fats
- Inositol, a type of alcohol
- Lignin
- The minerals calcium, iron, manganese, phosphorus, and potassium
- Resin
- Starch
- Sugar
- Vitamins A, C, and E

Dosing instructions and availability

Goldenseal is available through health food stores and drugstores in a variety of forms. Use a source that guarantees goldenseal content —other herbs have been found mixed into some products. Follow the dosage instructions on the bottle for its proper use. Common doses include 500 mg of dried root per day, and 1 dropperful of tincture 2–3 times per day. The dried herb may be made into a tea to treat all internal symptoms or to use as a mouthwash. Powdered goldenseal may be mixed with water to form a paste to externally treat warts or skin conditions such as chicken pox. Some people even put a capsule directly on a mouth sore to treat it.

Cautions

Goldenseal is generally considered safe. However, douches may cause irritation. Doses higher than recommended may cause nausea and vomiting. As with prescription antibiotics, your body may become immune to goldenseal's effects. It is generally recommended that you use goldenseal only when needed and then alternate the use of goldenseal with other natural antibiotics such as echinacea.

Added benefits

The list of benefits of goldenseal is a long one but well worth the time spent reading it. Benefits include:

- Cleanses the urinary tract
- Cleanses the lymph nodes
- Fights any infections, including acne
- Reduces nasal congestion and mucus production due to colds or allergies
- Helps soothe and heal wounds, including first- or second-degree burns
- Helps heal cold sores and mouth/throat irritations
- Relieves the itching of chicken pox while helping to prevent infection
- Helps lower blood pressure
- Increases the effectiveness of insulin
- Strengthens the immune system
- Detoxifies the body
- Stimulates the spleen, liver, colon, and pancreas
- Helps control acute diarrhea that is caused by intestinal bacterial infections
- Soothes and heals sore throats
- Stops excessive bleeding, including that of nosebleeds
- Soothes ulcers
- Heals warts
- Used in combination with echinacea, licorice, lemon balm, and ginger to fight chronic fatigue syndrome

Licorice

Glycyrrhiza glabra

Licorice is a shrub with spreading roots and rhizomes. It is native to subtropical areas, including Southeast Europe and Southwest Asia.

The basics of licorice

Licorice has a long history of medicinal use, dating from the Greeks, who used licorice for various respiratory illnesses, including asthma and coughs. Currently, licorice is often found as an ingredient in cough lozenges.

Alexander the Great also found good uses for licorice. His troops were sent out with a supply of licorice, among their other battle gear. The purpose? Troops were to chew their licorice sticks to alleviate their thirst, while also increasing their energy levels.

Licorice may help relieve symptoms of PMS and menopause because of its imitation of the effects of estrogen and progesterone and its anti-inflammatory properties.

Parts used

The root of the licorice plant is used.

Chemical content

Licorice contains these substances:

- Asparagine and choline, two amino acids
- Fat
- Glycyrretenic acid, a cough suppressant

- Glycyrrhizin and liquiritin, steroidal substances with antibacterial and anti-inflammatory properties
- Gum
- Inositol, a type of alcohol
- Lecithin
- The minerals manganese and phosphorus
- Pentacyclic terpene, a solvent-like substance found in the essential oil
- Proteins
- Sugars
- Vitamins B_1, B_2, B_3, B_6, and E

Dosing instructions and availability

This herb is added to many candies found in grocery stores. Health food stores and herb shops carry the licorice herb and teas containing it, as well as powdered root and liquid and solid extract. Other products containing licorice (such as cough suppressants) may be found in drugstores. Check ingredients lists on the labels—often anise is used instead of licorice as a flavoring for "licorice" candy.

Eat licorice sticks or foods prepared with licorice as an ingredient. For teas and other forms of licorice, follow product instructions. Common doses include 1–2 grams powdered root, 2–4 ml liquid extract, 250–500 mg solid extract, each taken 3 times per day.

Cautions

If you are pregnant; if you have diabetes, glaucoma, heart disease, high blood pressure, or severe menstrual problems; or if you have suffered a stroke, you should not use licorice without first consulting your healthcare provider. Even if you do not suffer from the above illnesses, you should not use licorice for more than 4–6 weeks at a time. Licorice has the potential to cause high blood pressure, swelling, high sodium levels, and low potassium levels.

Added benefits

Licorice has many other positive effects on the human body. For example, licorice contains glycyrrhizin, which kills bacteria, making licorice a wonderful tooth decay preventative. Here are other uses for licorice:

- Sexual stimulant
- Stimulates the production of interferon, which may be helpful to those with immune disorders
- Cleanses the colon
- Decreases muscular spasms
- Helps adrenal gland function
- Relieves respiratory diseases, such as asthma and emphysema
- Helps fight chronic fatigue syndrome
- Fights depression and stress
- Fights fever
- Helps fight hypoglycemia by raising blood sugar levels to normal levels
- Helps fight arthritis
- Normalizes ovulation
- Fights sore throats

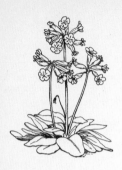

Primrose or Cowslip

Primula veris

This cool-loving plant grows 4–8 inches high and produces clusters of bright green leaves with yellow, fragrant flowers in early spring.

The basics of primrose

This herb has been used for centuries in Europe as a mild sedative and for respiratory problems. In addition, menopausal symptoms, such as hot flashes, may be alleviated by primrose. Women who suffer from many premenstrual symptoms, especially heavy cramps and heavy bleeding, should also benefit from using primrose. Although little is known about how this herb works, primrose is considered to be a natural estrogen promoter, which helps explain its ability to reduce menopausal and premenstrual symptoms. It also contains steroidal substances that serve as anti-inflammatories, which may also help provide relief of these symptoms.

Parts used

Dried roots and rhizomes and flowers are used medicinally.

Chemical content

Primrose contains many substances, including the following:

- Gamma-linolenic acid (GLA) and linoleic acid, which may be helpful for maintaining heart health
- Tannins, astringents used for healing skin problems

- Saponins, substances in the roots that may help lower blood pressure and have anti-inflammatory and anti-pain properties
- Flavonoids, which have antispasmodic and anti-inflammatory properties

Dosing instructions and availability

Primrose is available in many health food stores. It takes the form of dried flowers, extract, syrup, and tincture and can be found in herbal teas and cough preparations. A common dosage is 1–2 ml extract up to 3 times per day. Follow product instructions for proper dosage.

Cautions

Not much is known about the safety of primrose. Some people notice stomach problems and nausea after using the root. Others have noted skin irritation when handling primrose flowers.

Added benefits

Primrose is an excellent source of unsaturated fats, which may help reduce blood pressure while alleviating any skin disorders that you may have. Other benefits from taking primrose include:
- Reduces blood pressure
- A good remedy for laryngitis, bronchitis, colds, and coughs
- Alleviates skin conditions, including eczema and skin dryness
- Used to treat alcoholism
- May help in weight loss
- Used in the treatment of colitis
- May relieve the pain and stiffness of arthritis

Red Raspberry

Rubus idaeus

Raspberries produce delicious red berries on tall, thorny stems with clusters of tooth-edged leaves. This perennial is native to many places throughout the world.

The basics of red raspberry

For centuries in places as diverse as Greece and North America, red raspberry leaves have been used for many medicinal purposes, including stomach and skin problems, as well as a range of "female" problems. This herb, along with peppermint in a tea, is still used to help women who suffer morning sickness. Raspberry relaxes uterine muscles, helping to prevent false labor and making actual labor easier. It is also used to prevent hemorrhaging during labor. These same properties may help make red raspberry a good choice for relief of menstrual cramps while also regulating the flow of menstrual bleeding. However, studies have failed to identify the active substances, and results have been mixed.

Parts used

Bark, leaves, and roots of red raspberry are used. The leaves are considered most effective for treating morning sickness and PMS.

Chemical content

- Citric and malic acids
- Essential oils

- The minerals calcium, iron, magnesium, manganese, phosphorus, potassium, selenium, silicon, and sulfur
- Pectin, a type of fiber
- Tannic acid, a substance with astringent properties that soothe skin problems
- Vitamins B_1, B_3, C, D, and E

Dosing instructions and availability

Raspberry is available through health food stores in many forms for both internal and external use. It is also found in many herbal blends. For morning sickness and premenstrual problems, common doses are to drink up to 6 cups of raspberry tea per day or take 1–3 384 mg capsules 3 times per day.

Cautions

Red raspberry is generally considered to be safe, even in pregnant women.

Added benefits

Red raspberry is used by certain animal breeders to promote fertility in their male animals. Because of this, some believe that it may help increase fertility in men as well. Since red raspberry is relatively harmless, unless you are allergic, there would be no reason not to try it if you or your partner are experiencing infertility problems. Some other benefits of using red raspberry include:
- Because of its calcium content, red raspberry promotes healthier bones, teeth, and nails
- Heals canker sores and other mouth irritations
- A traditional treatment for diarrhea, safe even for children
- Relaxes intestinal spasms
- May increase the production of milk in nursing mothers

Rosemary

Rosmarinus officinalis

This perennial shrub with a distinctive aroma has long stems filled with needle-like leaves and produces tiny blue flowers.

The basics of rosemary

Rosemary has been used for centuries in Asia and Europe for a variety of ailments. Rosemary in olive oil massaged onto the scalp has long been thought to be a way to encourage hair growth. One of the original uses of rosemary was as a food preservative, primarily for meats. Rosemary is high in antioxidants, which help to prevent the fats in meats from spoiling.

Many women currently use rosemary as a method to alleviate menstrual cramps and promote menstrual flow. It also is used for calming nerves, anxiety, and irritability, symptoms often associated with PMS and menopause.

Parts used

Leaves, stems, and essential oil from flowers of rosemary are used.

Chemical content

- Bitters
- Borneol
- Camphene and camphor, which contribute to this herb's pungent smell
- Camosic acid
- Camosol

- Cineole, a nervous system stimulant
- Essential oils
- Pinene
- Resin
- Tannins

Dosing instructions and availability

Rosemary is available in many forms for internal and external use in grocery stores, health food stores, and drugstores. For an all-around pain reliever, add rosemary leaves or oil to your bath water. Common dosages for internal use include tea made from 4–6 grams of rosemary leaves per cup of water. Follow instructions on product labels for other forms of rosemary.

Cautions

Rosemary is generally considered safe. Oil should be used externally only. Pregnant women may want to avoid medicinal use of rosemary, since there is some possibility that it can cause contractions.

Added benefits

Rosemary is often called the "herb of remembrance" because of its ability to enhance your memory by improving circulation to your brain. Other benefits include:
- May help to prevent Alzheimer's disease
- May help to prevent aging
- Fights cataracts
- Rosemary essential oil is often used to treat depression
- Revives people who have fainted
- Fights bacteria
- Relaxes the stomach
- Stimulates circulation and regulates blood pressure

- Prevents liver toxicity
- May prevent cancers or tumors from starting
- Relieves pain, including that of headache
- Excellent weapon to fight body odor
- May help to prevent and treat wrinkles
- Relieves the pain and stiffness of arthritis
- Treats dandruff

Sage

Salvia officinalis

Sage can be found in many sizes, with a variety of flower colors. Common to all sage varieties are the long, slender leaves, usually gray-green in color, somewhat fuzzy, and aromatic. Most sage plants also grow spiky flowers.

The basics of sage

Sage seems to have an estrogenic effect on the body, which makes it ideal to use for premenstrual and menopausal symptoms; however, no studies have yet shown how or why sage is said to accomplish this action. Sage may reduce the intensity and duration of hot flashes, while alleviating the sweating associated with them. It may also ease other symptoms, such as vaginal itchiness and dryness, associated with menopause, including menopause induced by hysterectomy. Dysmenorrhea, or painful periods, is often relieved by using sage.

For vaginal itching, try using sage in a douche. Sage contains anticandida compounds, which make it an excellent douche for vaginal itching or infection.

Nursing mothers who are weaning their infants from breast milk often use sage to help dry up their milk.

Parts used

Leaves are generally used. A volatile oil is also made from the stems of sage.

Chemical content

- Camphor, which contributes to sage's characteristic aroma
- Flavonoids
- Resin
- Salvene
- Saponins
- Tannins, an astringent that soothes skin problems
- Terpene
- Thujone, a toxic substance that can cause convulsions and even death
- Volatile oils, which may help with digestive disorders

Dosage instructions and availability

Sage is available at grocery stores, health food stores, and drugstores. You can find it fresh or dried, as well as in extract, tincture, paste, and plaster forms. Follow product instructions for appropriate dosage.

Cautions

Generally, sage is considered safe when used in food, since cooking probably destroys most of the volatile oil. Sage oil itself is considered toxic and should not be taken internally. Otherwise, follow product instructions carefully; high levels of thujone, a substance contained in sage, may cause convulsions or seizures. Do not use sage at all if you currently suffer from a seizure disorder. Sage also may interfere with iron absorption, so increase your iron intake if using sage. Do not use if you are a nursing mother, and not trying to wean from it since sage may decrease your milk supply. You may also want to avoid medicinal use of sage if you are pregnant, since its estrogen-like effects are still under study.

Added benefits

Sage has a long-standing reputation as being good for the hair. Massaged into your scalp, it may help prevent hair loss. Added to shampoo, sage may help your hair retain its original color longer. And some folks with silver or gray hair report good results using sage to give their hair more luster and sheen. You may find many commercially prepared hair products on the market that contain sage, or you can simply add sage to your own shampoos. Some other benefits of using sage are:

- May help prevent and treat Alzheimer's disease, because sage inhibits an enzyme that breaks down acetylcholine, which seems to prevent this disease
- Stimulates the central nervous system
- Stimulates the digestive system
- Reduces sweating and salivation
- Contains tannins, which are used to treat mouth and throat irritations and disorders
- Sage oil rubbed onto the abdomen muscles during the last three weeks of pregnancy may help prepare and tone the muscles for delivery
- May contain antioxidants, which have a range of beneficial effects on the body

Sarsaparilla
Smilax officinalis

Sarsaparilla is a prickly, climbing, perennial plant with long, creeping roots. Sometimes it is referred to as Chinese root. Sarsaparilla is native to the Caribbean.

The basics of sarsaparilla

In the past, sarsaparilla was used by American Indian women as a tea drunk after childbirth to help expel the placenta. It is thought that the Crees used sarsaparilla in the treatment of syphilis. Sarsaparilla contains a testosterone-like substance that may be what causes it to increase sexual drive in men.

Sarsaparilla alleviates premenstrual symptoms and menopausal symptoms, including mood swings and irregular menstrual cycles. This effect may be due to the rather high content of steroid-like substances in sarsaparilla.

Parts used

The rhizome (roots) of sarsaparilla is used.

Chemical content

Sarsaparilla contains these ingredients:
- The minerals copper, iron, manganese, sodium, sulfur, and zinc
- Essential oils
- Fatty acids, including sitosterol and stigmasterin
- Glycosides, derivatives of sugars

- The chemicals parillin and sarsaponin
- Resin, an amber-colored sticky substance
- Saponins, sarsapogenin, and smilagenin, steroidal substances
- Sugars
- Vitamins A and D
- The chemical parillin

Dosing instructions and availability

This herb is available in some beverages found primarily at health food stores. You may also find it as an extract or tincture. A common dose is ¼–½ teaspoon of the tincture 1 to 3 times per day.
Follow product label instructions.

Cautions

Sarsparilla is considered safe. However, doses greater than recommended amounts can cause stomach upset.

Added benefits

Other uses of this plant include the following:
- Increases energy
- Protects from radiation exposure
- Regulates hormone levels
- Acts as a diuretic
- Lowers blood pressure
- Helps clear up skin conditions, such as psoriasis, shingles, and eczema
- Acts as a laxative
- Relieves symptoms of inflammatory diseases like arthritis

Soy

Glycine max

A member of the legume family, soy is an annual with "hairy" leaves and produces tan, pea-like beans.

The basics of soy

This annual plant produces beans that probably have more uses than practically any other plant. For centuries, the Chinese used soybeans as a treatment for warts.

It is also believed that the added estrogen-like activity of soy may help a woman conceive during the "less fertile" years before menopause. The estrogen-like compounds help those women who suffer from endometriosis.

Many other premenstrual symptoms can also be relieved by eating soy—for example, uterine pain, cramps, and irritability. Vaginal dryness and vaginal irritability, often symptoms of menopause and two major causes of discomfort during sex, are alleviated by the consumption of soy. Soy works because of the phytoestrogens contained in the plant. Phytoestrogens bind with the cells' estrogen receptor sites, not allowing possibly more harmful estrogens to bind with those same receptors and causing damage. It would be wise to note that Asian women have a lower rate of breast cancer, osteoporosis, and bone fractures than Western women do. It is thought that the soy they consume on a regular basis is the reason for this.

Parts used

The bean of the soy plant is most commonly used.

Chemical content

Soy is high in two estrogen-like compounds, genistein and daldzein, which are called phytoestrogens.

Dosing instructions and availability

Soy is all around you at the grocery store and the health food store. Soy comes in many edible forms: soy sauce, tofu (soy bean curd), soy milk, roasted soy nuts, and textured soy used as meat substitutes. You may also be able to purchase soy powder or soy tablets through health food stores. To achieve noticeable effects, you may need to consume a lot of soy products, such as several cups of soy milk per day. You may want to consult an herbalist to determine the level of soy that would best meet your needs.

Cautions

Few side effects of soy are noted. However, some people have allergies to soy products and should avoid this herb.

Added benefits

It is believed that the added estrogen benefits of soybeans help protect from heart disease. While using soy, you may also find yourself gaining relief from dandruff. Soy contains biotin, which is an enemy of dandruff.

How about getting rid of, or preventing, cold sores or shingles? Soy contains a high level of lysine, which is an amino acid that helps fight and prevent the outbreaks of cold sores and shingles.

Squaw vine

Mitchella repens

This herb is a ground-hugging evergreen vine with bright red berries that have little taste and stony seeds.

The basics of squaw vine

Squaw vine has traditionally been used as a uterine tonic. American Indian women used squaw vine for any purpose that would be associated with childbearing. During the final stages of pregnancy, they would drink tea made from squaw vine to strengthen the uterus and ensure an easy and safe delivery.

Currently, there may be those who still use squaw vine for this purpose. But it is known for easing menstrual pain, irregularities, cramps, anxiety, and irritability, though there is no formal study available that supports these uses.

Nursing mothers may want to take note that American Indian women also used squaw vine to treat nipple soreness created by their nursing infants. This can be accomplished by boiling 2 ounces of squaw vine in one pint of water. Add one pint of heavy cream. Boil down until it reaches the constituency of a salve. Apply when cooled to nipples and after each feeding session.

Parts used

Leaves and stems of squaw vine are used.

Chemical content

Squaw vine contains the following substances:

- Alkaloids
- Glycosides
- Tannins

Dosing instructions and availability

Squaw vine is available through health food stores as extract, as tincture, and in herbal blends. A common dose is 4 ml of extract taken daily. Follow product instructions for appropriate dosage levels.

Cautions

Not much is known about the safety of squaw vine. Pregnant women may want to avoid this herb, since it is associated with uterine contractions.

Added benefits

Although most of the benefits derived by squaw vine are women-oriented, squaw vine's sedative and tranquilizing properties may benefit others, too, in the following ways:
- Muscle spasms may be alleviated
- The inflammation of hemorrhoids may be relieved
- Wounds and other skin conditions may heal faster
- Anxiety may be reduced
- Squaw vine is also known for its sedative and tranquilizing effects

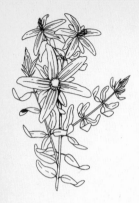

St. John's Wort

Hypericum perforatam

This perennial shrub has oblong leaves and bright yellow flowers. While native to Europe and Asia, St. John's wort can be grown in many parts of North America, where it is often considered an invasive weed.

The basics of St. John's wort

This herb's name comes from the fact that it used to be harvested on St. John's Day. St. John's wort is an old English plant used to treat depression and anxiety. There are studies that show St. John's wort to be more powerful in the treatment of depression and anxiety than many prescription medications, but with fewer side effects.

Some users of St. John's wort for anxiety or mood swings may find relief within a few days. However, realistically, it takes at least a couple of months to notice the effects of the herb. St. John's wort may also help relieve some of the symptoms of menopause, especially vaginal dryness, enabling you to enjoy sex more. This herb has also traditionally been used as a diuretic, which may make it helpful for relieving the bloating often associated with PMS. St. John's wort has also been used for relieving menstrual cramping, perhaps due to its sedative effects.

Parts used

Flowers, leaves, and stems of the St. John's wort plant are used.

Chemical content

The active ingredient that is responsible for St. John's wort's anti-depressive effects is hypericin, which is also being studied for use in fighting viruses such as AIDS. St. John's wort also includes tannins and other substances that may help fight infection.

Dosing instructions and availability

You can find this herb in most drugstores and health food stores. It usually comes as a pill, extract, oil, or tincture. It may also be available as an ointment for external use. Follow the labeling instructions carefully. A common daily dose is 0.2 to 1.0 mg hypercin per day, which translates into about 300 mg of capsules or extract.

Cautions

Do not use St. John's wort at the same time as using a prescription antidepressant, as it will exacerbate the effects on your body. Watch for increased sensitivity to light, both by your eyes and skin. Do not use while pregnant. Avoid wine and other alcohol, cheese, smoked or pickled foods, and some medications, even over-the-counter ones, taken to treat colds or hay fever. Also avoid amphetamines, narcotics, tryptophan, and tyrosine.

Added benefits

St. John's wort helps to promote sleep or even more restful sleep and boosts the levels of dopamine in the brain, which may reduce the risk of Parkinson's disease.

St. John's wort promotes the growth of tissue, which allows for less scarring from injuries and also helps to repair skin after a burn or other injury.

Some healthcare providers recommend the use of St. John's wort to treat bedwetting and nightmares in children.

Here are some other benefits associated with St. John's wort:

- Strengthens the immune system
- Acts as an expectorant
- Helps to heal bruises, strains, sprains, wounds, and muscle aches
- May help you to resist viral infections, including herpes

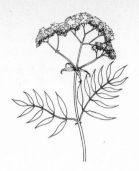

Valerian

Valeriana officinalis

This herb sports tall stems with rich, dark-green leaves and light colored flowers.

The basics of valerian

Another name by which valerian is known is "all-heal." This is a description of valerian's reputation as an antidote for just about everything. Ancient Romans used valerian to treat heart conditions, primarily heart arrhythmias and palpitations. Valerian is thought to be heart-healthy by increasing the blood flow and circulation, which allows the heart to pump better and more efficiently. This permits better blood flow to other areas of the body, including the genital areas.

Valerian's mild sedative and tranquilizing effect on the body relieves premenstrual symptoms such as nervous tension, irritability, cramps, and anxiety. However, no one has yet been able to establish how valerian accomplishes these effects.

Parts used

Roots and rhizomes of valerian are used.

Chemical content

- Acetic, butyric, and formic acids
- Camphene
- Chatinine

- Essential oils
- Glycosides
- Magnesium
- Pinene
- Valeric acid
- Valerine

Dosing instructions and availability

Valerian is available at health food stores in extract and capsule forms. Because it has the reputation of smelling like "dirty gym socks" and pretty much tastes like them too, you may prefer to take this herb by capsule form. A common dose is three 456 mg capsules taken 3 times per day.

Cautions

Valerian is generally considered safe. Because of its sedative effects, avoid taking this herb when driving or operating machinery.

Added benefits

Valerian is sometimes called an "herbal tranquilizer." And no wonder: it has sedative and tranquilizing powers, plus is considered to be one of the best sleep aids around! In the United Kingdom, over 80 sleep aids available without a prescription contain valerian as the active ingredient. And better yet, valerian is not considered to be habit-forming and doesn't leave you feeling all groggy and sleepy in the morning. But there are many other potential benefits to using valerian, too:

- Improves blood circulation throughout the body
- Reduces mucus and helps treat colds and allergies
- Reduces high blood pressure
- Relieves muscle cramps

- Alleviates the pain of ulcers
- Relieves tension
- Relieves irritable bowels
- May be used externally on tumors, and is thought to reduce their size

Wild Yam

Dioscorea villosa

Wild yam is a perennial vine with heart-shaped leaves, green flowers, and potato-like tubers. This herb is native to North America.

The basics of wild yam

American Indians used to consume wild yams to relieve a variety of aches and pains, including labor pains during the childbirth process. This herb was also used by American slaves.

Wild yam can give vigor to sex—while also relieving other symptoms that may make sex less enjoyable. The alleviation of vaginal dryness is one of the most commonly found uses for wild yam. But it can also relieve other symptoms of menopause, including hot flashes.

Women who experience painful periods, ovarian or uterine pain, or simply the "normal" premenstrual symptoms, may all find some relief with wild yams. The natural estrogen-like substances and other hormonal-like substances contained in wild yam may help regulate hormonal levels and serve as anti-inflammatories and muscles relaxants, making sex more pleasurable. However, as yet there are no formal studies supporting the effectiveness of wild yam.

Parts used

The rhizomes and roots of wild yam are used.

Chemical content

Wild yam contains a naturally occurring plant steroid, called dioxgenin, which is a natural precursor to progesterone (one of the female hormones). Other ingredients include:

- Alkaloids, bitter substances that occur in seed plants
- The chemicals kioscin and steroidal saponins
- Phytosterols, fatty substances found in plants
- Starch
- Tannins

Dosing instructions and availability

Wild yam cream is available at health food stores and drugstores in the form of capsules, cream, drops, extract, powder, and tincture. A common dosage for internal use is ½ teaspoon of tincture twice a day, two 505 mg capsules daily, or 2–4 ml liquid extract daily. For external creams, follow product instructions. Some prescription creams also contain wild yam—follow the prescription instructions.

For best absorption, wild yam creams should also be applied to the thinner skin of the body, such as the chest, breasts, lower abdomen, inner thighs, inner arms, wrist, and neck. It can be applied to the vaginal area to alleviate vaginal itching and dryness.

Cautions

Wild yam is generally considered safe. However, because it may influence hormones, pregnant women and anyone undergoing hormone therapy should avoid this herb. When using wild yams as an external cream, keep in mind that the skin you are rubbing it on may become sensitive to it. Rotate the areas where you apply it.

Added benefits

Some other benefits of using wild yam include:

- Alleviates kidney stones

- Relieves gallbladder disorders by promoting the production of bile
- Helps to regulate blood sugar levels, alleviating hypoglycemia
- Relieves pain associated with arthritis

7

Controlling Health Conditions that Affect Sex

Many health conditions can affect your ability to enjoy sex. Some conditions such as arthritis make it painful to move during sex. Other health problems impair blood flow and nerve sensation, making sexual fulfillment difficult. We'll discuss six of the most common health conditions that affect sex:

- Arthritis
- Bladder infections
- Cardiovascular problems
- Depression
- Diabetes
- Muscle aches and spasms

Next, we'll describe herbs that can help these conditions.

Arthritis

Many people suffer from arthritis, which can make joints swollen and stiff, preventing you from moving easily—especially during activities like sexual intercourse. There are two types of arthritis: osteoarthritis and rheumatoid arthritis.

Osteoarthritis is more commonly referred to as "wear and tear" arthritis. It occurs as the cartilage and bones of joints are worn down due to misuse or overuse.

Rheumatoid arthritis is an immune system disease, and its causes are not well understood. It is thought that after some sort of viral infection, the body overreacts, attacking the tissues of the joints rather than the virus. As the joints are under attack, they become swollen and painful. In some cases, the attacks and inflammation can even spread into the muscles. There are also many other conditions associated with rheumatoid arthritis.

For both types of arthritis, herbs can help relieve inflammation and pain. The following are some herbs that may help: **alfalfa, bay, blue cohosh, cat's claw, cayenne (capsicum), celery, dandelion, feverfew, ginger, kava, licorice,** and **wild yam.**

Bladder Infections

Practically everyone gets a bladder infection once in a while. If you have infections frequently, you may find that it interferes with your sex life. If you do have frequent bladder infections, you should see your doctor to treat the infection and to ensure there is no serious underlying cause. In addition, these herbs may help: **bilberry, birch leaves,** and **hydrangea.**

Cardiovascular Problems

Problems in the cardiovascular system take many forms: high blood pressure, heart disease, circulation problems in the legs. Most cardiovascular problems occur because of the buildup of plaque in the arteries, the blood vessels that carry oxygen-rich blood throughout the body. The arteries may also narrow and become less flexible for other reasons, such as aging, use of tobacco, or high blood pressure. When arteries become narrowed and less flexible, blood cannot flow freely to nourish parts of the body. This can cause problems throughout the body, such as heart attacks, strokes, and circulation problems in your legs. Another result of cardiovascular problems may be a lack of blood flow to those "private parts," both the female and male genitalia, inhibiting your ability to enjoy sex. For any cardiovascular problem, you should be under the care of your doctor. But check with your doctor to see if you might try some of these herbs to help you enjoy sex more: *alfalfa*, *bilberry*, *cayenne (capsicum)*, *celery*, *garlic*, and *mistletoe*.

Herbal Baths to Aid Circulation

These two herbal baths maintain and improve blood flow to the heart and other vital parts! Try a combination of marigold, nettle, and bladder wrack. Or use ginger. For either bath, simply place the herbs in a cheesecloth bag and let them soak in warm bath water with you.

Depression

Everyone gets the blues now and then. But depression can be a serious health threat—and can impinge on your ability to desire and enjoy sex. Depression can be caused by external events, but results in a chemical imbalance in the brain. Professional treatment can help. Some of these herbs may provide relief, as well: *dong quai*, *ginger*, and *St. John's wort*.

Diabetes

Some people develop diabetes when they are young, often after contracting a seemingly mild virus. In this "type I" diabetes, the body is unable to make insulin, a hormone that regulates the body's sugar (glucose) levels. Insulin shots must be taken to avoid death. Other folks develop diabetes as they age. People with "type II" diabetes usually have problems with their body's using the insulin that is made. They may need to take medication to control the condition. In both type I and type II diabetes, circulation problems and nerve damage may result, affecting your ability to enjoy sex. While controlling diabetes through diet, medication, and exercise is the key to mitigating complications such as impotence, these herbs may also provide some relief: *bilberry*, *dandelion*, and *garlic*.

Muscle Aches and Spasms

Do you have an occasional sore muscle from working (or playing) too hard? Or perhaps you have a serious medical condition such as multiple sclerosis that causes muscle spasms. In either case, muscle problems can inhibit your ability to enjoy sex. For serious health problems, you should be treated by a physician. But see if these herbal solutions also help: *catnip*, *licorice*, and *mistletoe*.

Alfalfa
Medicago sativa

This perennial bushy clover bears blue, purple, or yellow flowers.

The basics of alfalfa

Alfalfa was noted in 1597 by English herbalist John Gerard to be an herb capable of relieving an upset stomach. In the Arab world, they call alfalfa the "father of all herbs." It's no wonder, when you think of all the wonderful nutrients contained in alfalfa—eight essential amino acids, four times the amount of vitamin C as in a glass of citrus juice, and high levels of calcium.

Alfalfa helps maintain cardiovascular health, including regulating blood pressure and lowering cholesterol. Part of its action may be due to its diuretic effects, ridding the body of excess fluids. Saponin glycosides found in alfalfa leaves may help lower cholesterol levels, preventing plaque from building in the arteries. These substances may also have anti-inflammatory effects, helping to relieve pain associated with arthritis.

Parts used

The seeds, flowers, leaves, and sprouts of alfalfa are used.

Chemical content

Alfalfa contains these substances:
- Substances that act like estrogens in the body
- Alpha-carotene, a substance similar to beta-carotene (vitamin A)

- Chlorophyll, a green pigment
- Amino acids
- The minerals calcium, copper, iron, magnesium, phosphorus, potassium, sulfur, and zinc
- Saponin glycosides (in leaves), which may help lower cholesterol and prevent arterial plaque buildup as well as exerting anti-inflammatory effects
- Vitamins A, B-complex, C, D, E, and K

Dosing instructions and availability

You can easily grow alfalfa sprouts from seeds. Seeds and sprouts are readily available at most grocery and health food stores. Alfalfa is also available in pills, dried leaves, infusion, powder, and tincture forms.

For alfalfa pills, infusion, powder, and tincture, follow the instructions on the product label. Alfalfa sprouts can be added to sandwiches and salads.

Cautions

Contaminants have been found in some dried alfalfa products, so use a reputable source that guarantees contents. Alfalfa—especially the seeds—can cause systemic lupus erythematosus (SLE) to flare up in persons with this health condition.

Added benefits

Alfalfa aids in the relief from various "female" problems, namely menopausal and menstrual symptoms. It is also thought that alfalfa may increase the production of milk in nursing mothers, while also boosting the amount of vitamins contained in the milk.

Men who suffer from an enlarged prostate and increased urination due to this condition may also find relief with alfalfa. Alfalfa helps reduce the inflammation and swelling that occurs with this condition.

Other benefits of alfalfa include:

- Relieves constipation by giving you a healthy dose of fiber
- Relieves heartburn and indigestion by neutralizing acids
- Helps to prevent osteoporosis with its high calcium content
- Fights infections, including acne
- Purifies the blood
- May help prevent Alzheimer's disease by improving blood circulation to the brain
- The vitamin K contained in alfalfa is also thought to reduce morning sickness.
- High in chlorophyll, which makes for less body odor
- Natural source of fluoride for strong bones and teeth
- Aids in weight loss

Bay

Laurus nobilis

These evergreen, graceful trees with long, leathery leaves, clusters of small white flowers, and shiny black berries can be grown outdoors in warm-winter areas or in pots in cold-winter climates.

The basics of bay

Bay has long been used for many, mostly nonmedicinal, purposes. The Romans believed bay leaves could protect you from thunder and lightning, for example.

Medicinally, rubbing bay oil on painful joints may help relieve inflammation and pain. Perhaps this is due to its narcotic effects, essentially serving as a pain reliever.

Parts used

Leaves and an oil pressed from the seeds of bay are used.

Chemical content

Bay's essential oil, eugenol, has narcotic, sedative, bacterial, and fungicidal effects.

Dosing instructions and availability

Bay oil can be squeezed from seeds or purchased commercially. Bay leaves are available in the spice section of your grocery store. Bay oil can be rubbed onto the skin. Bay leaves can be used in cooking.

Cautions

Use caution when applying bay oil on your skin—it can cause dermatitis.

Added benefits

It has been used medicinally for many other reasons:
- Promotes menstruation
- Induces abortions
- Cures colds
- Repels insects

Bilberry

Vaccinium myrtyllus

This shrubby relative of the cranberry and blueberry has oval leaves and produces black berries.

The basics of bilberry

This shrub can be found in North America and Europe, where it has long been used to treat diarrhea and urinary tract infections. This benefit appears to come from the high tannin content of the dried berries. Other substances, anthocyanoides, are being studied to determine if they in fact can help improve blood oxygen supply and regulate blood sugar levels, which would benefit people with diabetes and circulation problems. Several small studies have supported potential benefit in these areas; other studies are underway.

Parts used

The berries (dried) and sometimes the leaves of bilberry are used medicinally.

Chemical content

Bilberry contains the following substances:
- Tannins, astringent substances
- Anthocyanoides, flavonoids that may boost the blood supply throughout the body

Dosage instructions and availability

Bilberry is available as capsules, drops, dried berries, powdered berries, and extract through herb shops and health food stores. A common dosage is to take two 500 mg capsules twice a day. For other forms, follow the instructions on the product label.

Cautions

Not much is known about the safety of bilberry; however, this herb has been used for centuries, with few side effects having been noted.

Added benefits

Bilberry has traditionally been used for a range of ills, including the following:

- Sores and inflammation in the mouth and throat
- Improvement of vision, especially night vision
- Peptic ulcers
- Varicose veins

Birch

various members of the Betula family

Birch is a deciduous tree or shrub generally recognizable by its smooth bark and usually has raindrop-shaped, jagged-edged leaves. There are about 40 different types of birch throughout the world.

The basics of birch

Birch has long been used by American Indians and Europeans. The medicinal use varies with the type of birch. For instances, Native Americans used a birch leaf tea for treating ailments ranging from fever to stomach upset. Europeans have used white and silver birch leaves to make a tea to soothe skin problems and as a diuretic. White or silver birch may help relieve urinary problems by causing you to urinate more, thus ridding the body of accumulated infectious organisms. This last use has some support from research.

Parts used

Leaves of birch are used medicinally, either as dried leaves or as an oil extracted from them.

Chemical content

Birch contains the following substances:
- Flavonoids
- Volatile oils that may serve as a diuretic
- Methyl salicylate, a substance similar to aspirin that relieves pain and inflammation

- Betulin, a substance that may prevent the spread of skin cancers

Dosing instructions and availability

Birch leaf tea is available in health food stores and herb shops. European white birch tar oil is also available through these same sources for external use. A common dose of the tea is 1–2 tablespoons of leaves per cup of water taken several times per day. Don't use boiling water, as it can destroy the volatile oil.

Cautions

Persons with heart or kidney problems should avoid birch tea. Birch tar oil can irritate the skin and cause kidney irritation when used for a long time or over much of the body. Birch tar oil contains high levels of methyl salicylate, which can be poisonous, especially in children, if taken internally.

Added benefits

Birch can provide additional health benefits:
- Treatment of skin problems such as eczema
- Possible relief of irritated joints
- Possible use in anticancer therapy

Blue Cohosh

Caulophyllum thalictroides

Blue cohosh is an herb that grows 12–30 inches in height, with a spread of just over 1 foot. Native to North America, blue cohosh likes low, rich, moist soil in swamplands or close to running water. Like black cohosh, blue cohosh is gathered from the wild. It is feared that the plant will become endangered before too long.

The basics of blue cohosh

Blue cohosh was used by the North American Indians primarily to relieve the symptoms of menstrual cramps, but also to help along childbirth, even to induce labor.

Steroidal substances in blue cohosh may help relieve pain and inflammation, such as that caused by arthritis or even routine muscle aches, allowing you to better enjoy sex.

Parts used

The roots of blue cohosh are used.

Chemical content

Blue cohosh contains these ingredients:
- The minerals calcium, iron, magnesium, phosphorus, potassium, and silicon
- Coulosaponin, a soapy, steroidal substance
- Gum
- Inositol, a type of alcohol
- The chemicals leontin and methylcystine

- Salts
- Starch
- B-complex vitamins and vitamin E

Dosing instructions and availability

This herb is available in pill and extract form through health food stores. Carefully follow the instructions on the product label or consult an herbalist.

Cautions

Since blue cohosh may help to facilitate and even to induce labor (the compound coulosaponin, which stimulates uterine contractions, is found in blue cohosh), it only makes sense *not* to use it during early pregnancy. Blue cohosh could cause miscarriage. It can also cause spasms of other muscles, such as the heart and intestines, which can be painful or even life-threatening. Eating leaves and seeds directly can cause stomach pain.

Added benefits

Other uses of blue cohosh include the following:
- Acts as a diuretic
- Acts as a uterine tonic
- Acts as a mild expectorant
- Helps to destroy or expel parasitic intestinal worms
- Produces or increases the production of perspiration, which may help in weight loss efforts or relief of edema
- Contains a steroid component, which helps to alleviate the symptoms of arthritis and common muscle aches
- May also alleviate the seizures of epilepsy
- Acts as an emmenagogue, which hastens menstrual flow

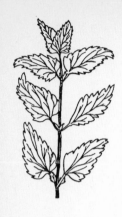

Catnip
Nepeta cataria

Spikes of small white flowers top stems bearing fuzzy, gray-green leaves with serrated edges. Catnip is a perennial that grows throughout the world.

The basics of catnip

The North American Indians used catnip as a sedative to calm nerves and to calm colic in young children. Because catnip contains chemicals that are similar to sedatives, it may be used to promote better or more restful sleep. Its mild tranquilizing effects also help calm nerves, stress, and anxiety. Catnip can even calm the stomach while aiding digestion, relieving pain, and preventing muscle spasms.

Parts used

Catnip leaves are used.

Chemical content

Nepetalactone is a substance found in the essential oil of catnip that may have sedative properties.

Dosing instructions and availability

You can find catnip drops, capsules, extract, and tincture in health food stores. You may also be able to find catnip as an ingredient in tea. Tea can be made using 2 teaspoons dried catnip per cup of water. Drink 1–3 times per day. For all other forms, follow the instructions on the label.

Cautions

Catnip is generally considered safe.

Added benefits

Catnip drops have been used by many to curb their cravings for nicotine. To try this, buy a small bottle of catnip drops and place several drops on the back of your tongue. Have the flu? Catnip may help by reducing your fever. Have a problem with low weight or no or low appetite? Catnip is also known for its ability to stimulate the appetite. Yet another possible benefit of catnip is that it is thought to reduce the risk of cataracts as you age.

Cat's Claw

Uncaria tomentosa and u. guianensis

Cat's claw is a vine native to South America and Asia. It has twisting, woody stems and branches.

The basics of cat's claw

South American Indians have used this herb for centuries as a general cure-all. Its anti-inflammatory properties may help reduce symptoms such as pain associated with arthritis, as well as other inflammatory conditions. However, no study has yet pinpointed the active substances and how they work.

Parts used

The bark of cat's claw root is used medicinally.

Chemical content

Cat's claw contains the following substances:
- Alkaloids, which may stimulate the immune system
- Glycosides, chemicals that reduce inflammation

Dosing instructions and availability

Cat's claw is available through health food stores and herb shops. It can be found in capsule and extract forms. A common dosage is one to two 500 mg capsules 3 times per day.

Cautions

Cat's claw has been used for many years without reports of ill effects.

Added benefits

Cat's claw is being studied for other possible health benefits, including the following:
- Ability to prevent the body's cells from becoming cancerous (antimutagenic)
- An immune system stimulator, possibly useful for persons with AIDS
- Ability to lower blood pressure, blood cholesterol, and heart rate

Cayenne or Capsicum

Capsicum annuum

Cayenne is a tropical perennial shrub with long, podlike berries.

The basics of cayenne

Spicy food, ornamental pods, criminal deterrent—these are probably the first uses you think of for cayenne pepper. Cayenne made it into the European cuisine thanks to Christopher Columbus's trips to the Americas. It has grown for centuries in other areas as well. Cayenne was used by the Greeks, and its formal name, *capsicum,* means "to bite." Ayurvedic medicine, the traditional form of medicine used in India, considers capsicum to be one of the best medicines around.

But probably the best-known quality of cayenne is its ability to provide relief from arthritis pain. Capsaicin, which is an ingredient of cayenne, is often used in arthritis cream formulas. It provides heat to the affected area, while also acting as a pain reliever. Cayenne can reduce inflammation of arthritic joints, also lowering the pain. This allows you to move more freely and enjoy sex. Studies show that used externally, capsicum interferes with Substance P, a chemical believed to transmit pain impulses. Capsicum is known to aid in the absorption of other herbs, including those that affect sexual desire and pleasure. This increases their effectiveness in the body.

Parts used

Berries of the cayenne bush are used.

Chemical content

Cayenne has several active ingredients that have helpful benefits:

- Vitamins A and C
- Capsaicin, a powerful stimulant and anti-inflammatory
- Salicylate, an aspirin-like substance

Dosing instructions and availability

This herb is as close as your grocery store spice section. You can also find cayenne in pill or extract form at health food stores. Creams containing capsaicin are readily available in drugstores. Or you can make your own liniment by boiling 1 tablespoon of cayenne in 1 pint of cider vinegar. Bottle while still hot.

For relief of arthritis, apply cayenne externally. For internal use, follow instructions on the product label.

Cautions

Don't use cayenne if you have intestinal disorders. It can make these conditions worse. Also, prolonged contact with the skin can cause blistering. Keep cayenne out of your eyes (wear rubber gloves when working with it).

Added benefits

Capsicum is thought to be a strong stimulant and a powerful tool for those who are trying to overcome an addiction to alcohol.

Capsicum is also heart-healthy. It cleanses and nourishes the blood vessels, while also strengthening the artery walls. It also discourages the formation of blood clots, which may lead to strokes or heart attacks. Capsicum also helps to lower the amount of cholesterol in the blood stream.

Weight loss may be easier when using capsicum. It promotes perspiration and increases thermogenesis, which is the production of heat in the body.

Other external and internal uses for the pepper abound:

- Relieving gas and diarrhea
- Easing symptoms of asthma
- Reducing pain of toothaches and sore throats
- Lowering fever

Celery

Apium graveolens

Celery is also sometimes called garden celery or wild celery. Either should work for these purposes. You're probably familiar with how celery looks when you buy it in the store: long, bright green stalks grown tightly together with delicate green leaves on top. If celery remains in the ground for a second year, it also develops small flowers that produce seeds.

The basics of celery

In Asian folk medicine, celery was used for hundreds of years to lower blood pressure, to improve circulation, and to eliminate or alleviate dizziness.

Celery may also help to alleviate symptoms of arthritis, possibly because of its ability to increase blood flow to inflamed areas.

Parts used

The root, stalk, seeds, and juice of the celery plant may be used.

Chemical content

Celery contains these substances:
- Apigenin, a chemical that relaxes the muscles that line the blood vessels, dilating the vessels and allowing the blood to pass through normally
- B-complex vitamins
- Iron
- Vitamins A and C

- Phthalides, substances that act as sedatives and anticonvulsants

Dosing instructions and availability

Celery is available in several forms:
- Fresh, on the stalk
- Root
- Seeds
- Oil from celery seeds
- Extract made from celery seeds
- Juice

Fresh celery, seeds, and dried leaves are readily available at your supermarket. Oil and extract (made from the celery seed) and juice may be found in health food stores. You can even make your own juice with fresh celery. Use celery in recipes and for snacks. Tinctures or infusions made from seeds are usually taken ½ to 1 teaspoon 1 to 3 times per day.

Cautions

Don't use celery as more than a food during pregnancy because of its ability to stimulate the uterus and cause miscarriage. Some people also develop skin reactions when handling celery. Its diuretic properties could harm persons with certain types of kidney disease.

Added benefits

Celery has also been used to treat loss of desire or low sexual drive in women. There are plenty of other benefits to eating celery:
- Acts as a diuretic
- Used as a general feel-good tonic
- Has a calming effect and works as a sedative, promoting sleep and more restful sleep

- Contains butylidenephthalide, a chemical that helps start menstrual flow
- Eliminates uric acid
- Lowers blood pressure and improves blood circulation
- Acts as a uterine stimulant; may help to facilitate childbirth
- Helps with weight loss by promoting perspiration
- Helps the kidneys and liver function properly, which increases urine flow
- Used to assist the digestive process; contains fiber
- Helps to balance the body's chemicals, which may help with illnesses involving chemical imbalances

Cranberry

Vaccinium macrocarpon

This evergreen shrub thrives in cool, boggy areas of North America and produces large, bright red berries.

The basics of cranberry

From several generations of Native Americans to modern physicians, practically everyone promotes cranberry juice as a treatment for urinary tract infections. Several studies support these claims, though how cranberries accomplish this cure remains unknown.

Parts used

The berries of the cranberry bush are used medicinally.

Chemical contents

Cranberries contain a lot of vitamin C. The substances that contribute to this berry's medicinal properties, however, are still being identified.

Dosing instructions and availability

Cranberry juice is readily available in grocery stores, usually in the form of juice cocktail, with sweeteners (a huge amount!), water, and sometimes other juices added. A common dose to prevent urinary tract infections is 3 ounces of cranberry juice cocktail taken daily. A common dosage to treat urinary tract infections is 12–32 ounces taken each day.

Cautions

Cranberry juice is generally considered safe. However, if a urinary tract infection persists or recurs frequently, you should seek medical attention to identify and treat the underlying cause.

Added benefits

Cranberry juice is often also used to treat another urinary tract problem, cystitis, and to deodorize the urine.

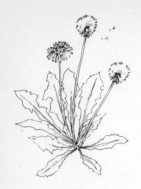

Dandelion

Taraxacum officinale

Dandelion is native to Europe, but now grows wild throughout the world. This short perennial produces long, grooved leaves and bright yellow flowers.

The basics of dandelion

Dandelions are full of vital nutrients, including potassium. European herbalists have used it for centuries to treat diabetes, liver diseases, and anemia.

People with diabetes are more likely to have difficulty with sex, because of a lack of blood flow and nerve damage associated with the disease. Dandelion has been shown to lower blood sugar levels in animals, and may also help people with diabetes achieve stable blood sugar levels. Maintaining a good blood sugar level may also reduce food cravings in those who wish to lose some weight. Substances in the root may also reduce inflammation—good news for people with arthritis.

Parts used

Dandelion leaves, roots, and flowers are used.

Chemical content

Dandelion contains these ingredients:
- Bioflavonoids, substances similar to vitamins
- The minerals calcium, iron, magnesium, phosphorus, potash, sulfur, and zinc

- Choline, an amino acid
- Gluten
- Inositol, a type of alcohol
- The chemicals lactupierine and linolenic acid
- Resin
- Sesquiterpene lactones and taraxacin, bitter substances that stimulate appetite and aid digestion
- Vitamins A, B_1, B_2, B_6, B_{12}, C, and E

Dosing instructions and availability

It's probably all around you. You can use dandelion greens and roots fresh from the ground, but be sure you don't pick them from an area that has been treated with chemicals (pesticides, insecticides, herbicides, or fertilizer). Dandelion may also be available as capsules, dried flowers, root juice, powdered root, tincture, or extract in health food stores or herb shops. Use fresh, young greens in salads. For products containing dandelion, follow label instructions carefully. Common dosages are 1–2 teaspoons of tincture 1–3 times per day or 1 tablespoon juice in water 2 times per day.

Cautions

Dandelion is generally considered safe.

Added benefits

Dandelion is thought to be one of the best natural diuretics, making it an excellent way to detoxify your body and to lose weight. Others suggest its use for treatment of urinary tract infections. Dandelion also reduces the amount of uric acid, which helps the elimination and prevention of kidney stones.

Dandelion also is used in the treatment of liver problems. Dandelion helps to promote the flow of bile from the liver. It also may help those suffering from hepatitis, cirrhosis, and jaundice.

Others believe that dandelion may help to prevent breast cancer in some women. The juice from the dandelion stem may also be used directly on a wart to dry it up.

Dong Quai
Angelica sinensis

This perennial has purple stems, clusters of white flowers, and thick, branched roots.

The basics of dong quai

Dong quai is often called "the woman's herb," but it has many other uses as well. Records as far back as 588 B.C. show dong quai recommended for the treatment of painful menstrual cycles. In both China and Japan, dong quai has long held a reputation as "women's ginseng" and is second in sales only to licorice root. Its Latin name, *Angelica,* comes from the legend that its healing powers were revealed in a dream. An angel supposedly told the dreamer that it was a cure for the plague. Dong quai also used to be known as the "root of the Holy Ghost."

Some persons suffering from mild depression, anxiety, or stress may find relief in using dong quai, allowing them to enjoy sex more. Dong quai acts like a sedative and has a mild tranquilizing effect on those who take it. This herb may also help people with high blood pressure, as it contains many substances that may help lower blood pressure.

Parts used

Dong quai roots are used.

Chemical content

Dong quai contains several known ingredients, some of which can be harmful when used in purified forms. Ingredients include the following:

- Phytoestrogens, which act like estrogen in a woman's body
- Psoralen, bergapten, and other coumarin derivatives, which dilate blood vessels and relax muscles
- Safrole, a substance found in the essential oil, which in pure form can cause cancer

Dosing instructions and availability

Dong quai comes as a capsule, extract, powder, and in other forms. It is also included in some beverages marketed to enhance sexual pleasure. Often, it is an ingredient in Chinese soups. When taking the capsule, extract, powder, or other medicinal forms, follow instructions on the product's label. A common dose is 3–5 grams per day. Avoid purified forms of dong quai.

Cautions

Dong quai can cause miscarriage. Coumarin derivatives may cause sun sensitivity and cancer. Purified safrole can cause cancer.

Added benefits

Dong quai balances female hormones, alleviating the pain and frustration of menstrual cycles and menopause. Some women report an increase in breast size after using dong quai. Used after childbirth, dong quai is considered to be a postpartum tonic. Quite possibly one of the best uses for dong quai is as a vaginal lubricant.

Dong quai is even recommended for men. Besides acting like a sedative for men, it is sometimes used to prevent testicular diseases. Dong quai also has antibiotic qualities, quite possibly being able to keep you from getting sick. It is a blood builder, which helps to heal all wounds and treat those who suffer from anemia. It is a bowel lubricant, helping those who suffer from constipation. Other benefits of dong quai include the following:

- Enhances vitamin E activity in those who are deficient
- Relieves insomnia
- Nourishes the brain
- Relieves arthritis pain
- Acts as an expectorant to treat bronchial conditions or coughs
- Helps to relieve gas and indigestion
- By increasing estrogen levels, dong quai may be used in the treatment of infertility
- May stimulate the appetite

Feverfew
Tanacetum parthenium

Feverfew, a perennial plant, grows wild in North America and other places throughout the world as a two-foot tall, hedge-like plant with yellow, daisy-like flowers. This herb is also called featherfew and featherfoil.

The basics of feverfew

The word feverfew comes from the Latin word *febrifugia*, which translates to "driver out of fevers." Since the Middle Ages, this herb has been used for just that purpose. Currently, though, feverfew has been making quite a name for itself for its success in the treatment of headaches—not just any old headache, but migraine headaches. Feverfew's ability to relieve pain also makes it a useful herb for people with arthritis, allowing more pain-free movement so that sex may become more enjoyable.

Parts used

Bark, dried flowers, and leaves of feverfew are used.

Chemical content

- Bomeol
- Camphor
- Parthenolide, the primary substance believed responsible for pain relief
- Pyrethrins
- Santamarin

- Sesqueterpine lactones, chemicals that may have both antipain and antispasmodic properties

Dosing instructions and availability

Feverfew may be made into a tea; however, most will find it better to take feverfew in capsule or extract form. Feverfew leaves are known to have a not-very-pleasant taste, and may cause mouth sores and an inflammation of the tongue and mouth. It is generally recommended that you take 60–380 mg of the capsules or 4–8 ml of extract per day; however, concentrations of parthenolide vary from product to product, so follow the label instructions carefully.

Cautions

Feverfew is generally considered safe. The most common side effect is mouth ulcers. Pregnant women should never use feverfew. Because of its ability to cause uterine contractions, it could also possibly cause a miscarriage. It is also suggested that nursing mothers do not use feverfew. Feverfew may also affect drugs used to prevent clots, such as aspirin, heparin, and warfarin.

Added benefits

By taking feverfew on a regular basis, many migraine headache sufferers have been to reduce the number of headaches, while also reducing the severity of them. To find this relief, however, feverfew must be taken on a daily basis. It works as a preventative, and shouldn't just be taken when sufferers feel a migraine headache coming on.

Feverfew works to prevent migraines by inhibiting the production of prostaglandins, substances that are known to constrict and dilate blood vessels to the brain and may cause migraine headaches. One study shows that two-thirds of those who suffer from migraine headaches and were given feverfew were able to prevent migraine headaches.

Although best known for its headache relief, feverfew is often used as an all-around pain reliever. Here are some other benefits of using feverfew:

- Relief from allergies
- Relief of muscle pain and tension
- Stimulation of appetite
- Stimulation of uterine contractions
- Control of nausea

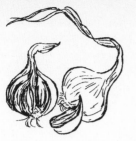

Garlic
Allium sativum

Onion-like stems bear purple blooms, while a large bulb made of many individual cloves forms underground on the garlic plant.

The basics of garlic

You may never regret eating too much garlic again—after all, this herb may help improve your sex life. One of the most valuable herbs around ever since biblical times is garlic. During the construction of the pyramids in Egypt, the builders used garlic to keep up their endurance and strength. In more recent times, during World War II, garlic was used as an antibiotic to treat wounds, infections, and even gangrene. Garlic is even known as "Russian penicillin" because of its antibiotic qualities.

A Japanese study showed that garlic may slow physiological aging and age-related memory loss in test animals. One study done in Pennsylvania indicated that garlic may help babies nurse better. Garlic was given to nursing mothers one hour before nursing. It was found that the nursing babies attached to the breast better, nursed longer, and drank more milk.

Garlic helps control blood sugar levels, so those who are diabetic or hypoglycemic may benefit from its use. It can also dilate the blood vessels, restoring blood flow to genital areas. Garlic aids blood flow and thins the blood by inhibiting platelet aggregation or clustering, which reduces the risk of blood clots and heart attack and may prevent migraine headaches from occurring. Garlic is also known for lowering cholesterol, which also helps to prevent heart attacks.

Parts used

The garlic bulb and its cloves are used.

Chemical content

Garlic contains many helpful substances, including:

- Alliin, an amino acid derivative that converts to allecin, which has antibiotic effects on the body
- Methyl allyl trisulfides, which dilate the blood vessels, allowing for proper blood flow throughout the body
- The minerals calcium, chromium, cobalt, copper, iodine, iron, magnesium, nitrogen, phosphorus, potassium, selenium, sodium, sulfur, and zinc
- Vitamins A, B_1, B_2, and C

Dosing instructions and availability

This herb is readily available in many forms. The produce section of your grocery store probably has fresh garlic bulbs and crushed, minced, and clove garlic in jars. Dried garlic can be found in the spice section. Garlic pills, including the odorless kind, are readily located in drugstores, health food stores, and mail order catalogs. You can easily grow garlic just by planting individual cloves. Garlic can be added to foods while cooking, or garlic pills can be taken by mouth. For garlic pills, follow the instructions on the label. Common doses of garlic include 1–5 fresh cloves daily or 10–20 grams of garlic extract daily.

Cautions

Besides strong breath and a garlic-like body odor, side effects from eating garlic are rare. They include nausea, vomiting, and diarrhea. Garlic may affect medications that lower blood sugar levels and thin the blood. Garlic can cause uterine contractions, so pregnant women should use this herb only as food.

Added benefits

The benefits for garlic seem to be endless—too many to include in this book. Garlic is a natural remedy for the following:

- Fever blisters
- Arthritis
- Aiding digestion
- An immune system stimulant
- Treating ulcers

Ginger
Zingiber officinale

This perennial produces spikes bearing purple flowers, with knotty roots and rhizomes forming underground.

The basics of ginger

Although ginger originated in Southeast Asia, the Spaniards introduced and naturalized ginger in America. In fact, ginger eventually became so popular with Europeans, that in 1884, 5 million pounds of ginger root was imported to Great Britain.

Many folks for years have sworn by using ginger for anxiety and depression. How ginger achieves this effect is as yet unknown. However, it is considered safe enough to even be used with other herbs taken for these purposes.

Parts used

The roots and rhizomes of ginger are used medicinally.

Chemical content

Ginger contains the following long list of substances:
- Acrid resin
- Bisabolene
- Bomeal and bomeol
- Camphene
- Choline
- Cineole
- Citral

- Gingerol, one of the main active ingredients, which prevents blood clotting
- Inositol
- The minerals manganese and silicon
- Phellandrene
- Sequiterpene
- B vitamins
- Zingerone
- Zingiberene

Dosing instructions and availability

Ginger root is available fresh, dried, powdered, candied and pickled in grocery stores and health food stores. It is also available in health food stores and herb shops as an extract or tea and in capsule and tincture form. Common dosages include 3–10 grams of fresh ginger per day, 2–4 grams of dried ginger per day, an inch square of candied ginger per day. For other forms, follow the product label.

Cautions

Using too much ginger may cause an stomach upset.

Added benefits

Those folks who suffer from migraine headaches are always looking for a better cure. Some people report that using ginger reduces the intensity and severity of their migraine headaches. Some other possible benefits you may get from using ginger include:

Relief from both morning sickness and motion sickness, or any other form of nausea—try one cup of ginger tea first thing in the morning or before driving/riding in a car, boat or other vehicle.

Relief from kidney pain; also promotes increased urine flow, allowing the kidneys to work more efficiently. Press hot compresses soaked in ginger tea to your lower back to alleviate kidney pain.

Ginger is considered to be an antiviral herb, which can help it combat many different conditions, including chronic fatigue syndrome and even sore throats

Ginger helps soothes an upset stomach due to indigestion; it contains chemicals that soothe the stomach and it keeps the food moving through the intestinal tract.

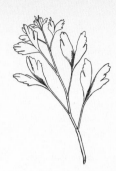

Ginkgo
Ginkgo biloba

This deciduous ornamental tree, native to China, has fan-shaped leaves and yellow seeds that give off a rather unpleasant odor.

The basics of ginkgo

Ginkgo is at times referred to as the "smart herb," because of its ability to enhance the memory and even possibly slow down the progression of Alzheimer's disease. Ginkgo doesn't perform miracles, but produces these effects by increasing blood flow throughout the body, enabling the user to feel stronger and more alert. By stimulating and improving blood circulation throughout the body, ginkgo provides more oxygen to the brain, heart, and all other body parts. It may help prevent heart attacks and other cardiovascular problems. Ginkgo's stimulating effects may also ease symptoms of depression, making you feel more energetic and desiring sex more.

Parts used

The leaves and nuts of the ginkgo tree are used.

Chemical content

- Gingko extract contains the active ingredients of flavone glycosides and terpenes.
- Gingkolides are steroidal substances in the tree currently under research.

Dosing instructions and availability

This herb is available in grocery, drug, and health food stores, as well as through herb shops and mail order companies. It comes in pills, extract, and added to products.

Follow the instructions on the product's label. It takes several months to begin to feel the effects of ginkgo. Many herbal practitioners believe that the amount of the active ingredients in ginkgo leaves are too diluted. To get enough ginkgo to be of much benefit, it is suggested that you take ginkgo in a standardized form, such as an extract or capsule. The usual dosing amount is 40 mg of extract 3 times per day or 60 to 240 mg in capsule form per day. Take this herb with meals to avoid stomach upset.

Cautions

Don't use more than 240 mg of ginkgo per day. Ginkgo can act as a blood thinner, so if you are already taking blood-thinning medication (including aspirin), avoid this herb. There have been reports of diarrhea, restlessness, and irritability when using ginkgo.

Added benefits

Take a look at what else ginkgo may do for you:
- Improve mental ability, such as memory, clarity, and alertness
- May slow down the advancement of Alzheimer's disease
- Provide relief from tinnitis, or ringing in the ears
- Relieve muscle aches and pains

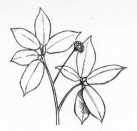

Ginseng

Panax ginseng, p. quinquefolius

A low-growing, shade-loving plant, ginseng produces red berries on stems surrounded by clusters of five leaves. The plant grows slowly, taking from two to five years for the root to be ready for harvest.

The basics of ginseng

Ginseng is an extremely expensive but wonderful herb that has been used medicinally for thousands of years. Its botanical name, *panax*, comes from a Greek word, *panacea*, which means "all healing." In China, it is sometimes referred to as the man's plant, referring to the shape of the ginseng root. Ginseng roots are considered to be more valuable because of their increased effectiveness as they age. The oldest roots available have been known to sell for as much as $20,000 per root! It is estimated that America, primarily the Northwest United States and Canada, exports some $100 million worth of American ginseng every year; 90 percent of this ends up in China. Ginseng is sometimes referred to as the herbal "Fountain of Youth."

Despite its widespread use, no one is sure yet how ginseng works. There have been studies done by Russian scientists showing that ginseng stimulates physical and mental activities and improves endocrine gland functions. Ginseng's effects on the endocrine glands may also make it helpful for controlling diabetes, thus helping to prevent complications of this disease that can inhibit sexual performance.

Parts used

The root of the ginseng plant is used.

Chemical content

Ginseng contains ginsenosides, steroidal substances that affect the central nervous system and help the body adapt to environmental and mental stress.

Dosing instructions and availability

This herb is easily available in powder, pill, and extract form at your grocery store, health food store, drugstore, or herb shop. You can also find ginseng added to many other food products and beverages that are marketed as increasing energy. Common doses are 1–2 grams of root per day or 250 to 1,000 mg of capsules. Amounts of ginseng vary considerably from product to product, so read labels and follow product instructions carefully. (See page 84 for information on the three kinds of ginseng.)

Cautions

Since ginseng is overharvested and expensive, some unscrupulous manufacturers substitute ingredients. Purchase products that guarantee their contents or buy ground ginseng root to avoid possible side effects from unknown substances.

Side effects from ginseng are rare, but include nervousness and diarrhea. Those suffering from hypoglycemia, diabetes, low or high blood pressure, or any heart disorder should closely monitor their symptoms when using ginseng. Also, women should not use ginseng in large amounts, or for too long, as it increases testosterone production, which is a male sex hormone, and may result in a lowering of the voice and increase of body or facial hair.

Drug interactions

Ginseng may also interact with certain types of medications, both over-the-counter and prescription. More specifically, some antibiotic, tranquilizer, sedative, and antihistamine medications may interact with ginseng, so always use with caution and read all labels.

Added benefits

There is a long, long list of other benefits that you may gain from the use of ginseng. There have been reports of some athletes using ginseng to enhance their athletic performance, while also increasing their endurance. Many athletes also use it for over-all body strengthening and conditioning as well. Others include:

- Fights fatigue, while acting as a stimulant
- Improves brain functions, such as memory, clarity, or alertness
- Helps heal the prostate gland
- Aids in the digestive process
- Reduces stress
- Strengthens and stimulates the adrenal glands and reproductive organs
- Stimulates appetite
- May help treat infertility
- Increases mental alertness
- Helps to lower blood pressure
- Helps to prevent heart disease
- Helps to condition the lungs, aiding in the treatment of emphysema, asthma, or chronic bronchitis
- Used to detoxify the body, aiding in the fight against addictions

Hydrangea

Hydrangea aborescens

A shrub growing to ten feet tall, hydrangea has woody stems with large, round leaves. Hydrangea produces clusters of white flowers. Note that this hydrangea is native to North America. It is not the same as those usually used as ornamentals. Nor is it the same hydrangea used in traditional Chinese medicine.

The basics of hydrangea

The name hydrangea is derived from a Greek word meaning "water-vessel." Hydrangea was once used by the Cherokee Indians as a diuretic and in the treatment of "calculi," that is, stones or deposits in the kidneys. It is still thought to be an excellent herb to purge the kidneys, as well as an overall tonic. Hydrangea root may help improve your sex life if you have frequent bladder infections that interfere with sexual enjoyment. Hydrangea helps to evacuate gravelly deposits from the bladder, alleviates the pain from passing deposits from the bladder, acts as a diuretic, and stimulates kidney function.

Part used

Only the roots of the hydrangea plant should be used.

Chemical content

Hydrangea contains these substances:

- Essential oils
- Saponin, a soapy substance

- Resin, a yellow, sticky substance

Dosing instructions and availability

This herb is available in pill and extract form from health food stores and herb shops. Follow the product label instructions.

Cautions

Do not use the leaves or buds of the hydrangea plant. They contain cyanide, and can be toxic. Too much hydrangea root may cause vertigo (dizziness) in some people.

Added benefits

Hydrangea also has the following uses:
- Helps correct bedwetting in children
- Helps treat obesity
- Acts as a laxative
- May be useful in treating allergies

Kava or Kava Kava

Piper methysticum

Kava is a large flowering shrub and a member of the pepper family of plants. The shrub produces knotty roots. It grows only in tropical forests, but its use in nontropical areas is booming.

The basics of kava

Many years ago, kava was "discovered" by the explorer Captain James Cook, who dubbed this herb "intoxicating pepper." Before Cook's discovery, however, the ancient Tahitians and other Pacific Islanders used—and continue to use—kava as a general all-around feel-good tonic and a stimulant.

Kava is known to be a good source of pain relief for those suffering from rheumatism. Kava may be used both externally and internally to treat all types of pain. It also serves as a muscle relaxant. All these effects of kava can help you remain pain-free, which can certainly help you enjoy sex more.

Kava's diuretic properties can also help relieve bladder problems.

Parts used

The kava root is used.

Chemical content

Kava contains two chemicals that are known to relieve pain: the kavalactones dihydrokavain and dihydromethysticin.

Dosing instructions and availability

Kava can be found in capsule, extract, powder, and root. It's best to use kava that has been prepared by a reputable supplements company, so that the active ingredients will be at a consistent level. Follow labeling instructions carefully.

Cautions

Kava is generally considered to be a safe and mild tranquilizer and an all-around tonic when used in small amounts (up to 250 mg of kavalactones daily). However, if you are already using a medication that has similar effects as kava, be careful! A few cases have been reported of people falling into a coma after combining kava with alcohol or antidepressant or antianxiety medications. Work with your doctor if you want to try kava in addition to or in place of these medications.

In addition, there is some evidence that kava may become addictive. Continuous use can lead to skin and blood problems. Avoid kava when you need to remain alert, such as for driving and operating machinery.

Added benefits

Kava is also considered to be one of the most powerful herbal muscle relaxants available today. In addition, it is good for calming nerves, fighting anxiety, and alleviating stress. Kava can also help put an insomniac to sleep while also enabling the user to obtain a more restful sleep.

Licorice

Glycyrrhiza glabra

Licorice is a shrub with spreading roots and rhizomes. It is native to subtropical areas, including Southeast Europe and Southwest Asia. Licorice grows as a spreading shrub and is native to Southeast Europe and Southwest Asia.

The basics of licorice

Licorice has a long history of medicinal use, dating from the Greeks, who used licorice for various respiratory illnesses, including asthma and coughs. Currently, licorice is still often found as an ingredient in cough lozenges.

Alexander the Great also found good uses for licorice. His troops were sent out with a supply of licorice among their other battle gear. The purpose? Troops were to chew their licorice sticks to alleviate their thirst, while also increasing their energy levels.

Licorice's anti-inflammatory properties may help relieve symptoms of arthritis, making sex less painful.

Part used

The root of the licorice plant is used.

Chemical content

Licorice contains these substances:
- Asparagine and choline, two amino acids
- Fat
- Glycyrretenic acid, a cough suppressant

- Glycyrrhizin and liquiritin, steroidal substances with antibacterial and anti-inflammatory properties
- Gum
- Inositol, a type of alcohol
- Lecithin
- The minerals manganese and phosphorus
- Pentacyclic terpene, a solvent-like substance found in the essential oil
- Proteins
- Sugars
- Vitamins B_1, B_2, B_3, B_6, and E

Dosing instructions and availability

This herb is added to many candies found in grocery stores. You can also find the herb and teas containing it in health food stores and herb shops, as well as powdered root and liquid and solid extract. Other products containing licorice (such as cough suppressants) may be found in drugstores. Check ingredient lists on the labels—often anise is used instead of licorice as a flavoring for "licorice" candy.

Eat licorice sticks or foods prepared with licorice as an ingredient. For teas and other forms of licorice, follow product instructions. Common doses include 1–2 grams powdered root, 2–4 ml liquid extract, 250–500 mg solid extract, each taken 3 times per day.

Cautions

If you are pregnant; have diabetes, glaucoma, heart disease, high blood pressure, or severe menstrual problems, or have suffered a stroke, you should not use licorice without first consulting your healthcare provider.

Even if you do not suffer from the above illnesses, you should not use licorice for more than 4–6 weeks at a time. Licorice has the potential to cause high blood pressure, swelling, high sodium levels, and low potassium levels.

Added benefits

Licorice has many other positive effects on the human body. For example, licorice contains glycyrrhizin, which kills bacteria, making licorice a wonderful tooth decay preventative. Here are other uses for licorice:

- Sexual stimulant
- Stimulates the production of interferon, which may be helpful to those with immune disorders
- Cleanses the colon
- Decreases muscular spasms
- Helps adrenal gland function
- Has estrogen- and progesterone-like effects
- Relieves respiratory diseases, such as asthma and emphysema
- Helps fight chronic fatigue syndrome
- Fights depression and stress
- Fights fever
- Helps fight hypoglycemia by raising blood sugar levels to normal levels
- Normalizes ovulation
- Fights sore throats

Marshmallow
Althaea officinalis

This perennial plant produces velvety leaves, large light-pink flowers, and long roots.

The basics of marshmallow

This is probably one of the oldest medicinal herbs, having been found in Neanderthal grave sites. It has been used for ills ranging from diarrhea to relieving sore throats. In fact, the sticky white fluffy stuff you toast in campfires originated as a meringue-sugar-marshmallow combination to give to children to soothe their sore throats. Modern-day marshmallows no longer contain this herb, however.

One traditional use of marshmallow has been to relieve kidney and bladder problems. This herb accomplishes this by serving as a diuretic, ridding the body of infectious organisms. It may also serve as an immune system booster, though how it accomplishes this benefit is not yet known.

Parts used

The root, leaves, and flowers of marshmallow are used medicinally.

Chemical content

Marshmallow contains mucilage, the substance that helps soothe irritated throats. Other substances in the herb are still being determined.

Dosing instructions and availability

Marshmallow is available at health food stores and herb shops as capsules, dried leaves, syrup, and tincture for internal use. It can also be found as a gargle, gel, ointment, or paste for external use. A common dose for internal use is 1 teaspoon of leaves per cup of water.

Cautions

Marshmallow is generally considered safe. It may cause other medications to be absorbed more slowly, however.

Added benefits

Marshmallow has other known and possible benefits, including the following:

- Protecting and soothing irritated skin and mucous membranes (mouth and throat)
- Helps suppress coughing
- May lower blood sugar levels
- May fight bacteria and boost the immune system
- May help with wound healing

Mistletoe
Viscum flavescens

You've probably seen the small green leaves and white berries of mistletoe hanging over doorways at Christmastime. In the wild, mistletoe takes root in the branches of oak and other trees.

The basics of mistletoe

Ever since the late 1600s, French herbalists have used mistletoe to treat a whole variety of ailments, including epilepsy, nervous disorders, and spasms. Mistletoe is still considered to be a stimulant for the heart, relieving symptoms of angina (chest pain) and irregular heartbeat (arrhythmia). Mistletoe also strengthens the capillary (small blood vessel) walls, helping to lower blood pressure.

If you have heart problems or high blood pressure that limit your ability to enjoy sex, mistletoe may help regulate these conditions.

Mistletoe also contains natural muscle relaxants, which may relieve muscle spasms or just make you feel better after a good workout.

Parts used

Mistletoe leaves and twigs are used.

Dosing instructions and availability

This herb is available at health food stores, usually as an infusion from leaves. Other forms such as capsules, injection, and extract are used in Europe, but are not available in the United States. Follow label instructions carefully.

Cautions

Mistletoe berries are considered to be highly poisonous in children. Avoid using mistletoe during pregnancy; it may cause uterine contractions and lead to miscarriage. Mistletoe may interfere with blood pressure medications.

Added benefits

Mistletoe is also considered to be a sedative, making it useful for headache sufferers. The mild tranquilizing effects it has may even help those who suffer from epilepsy to have fewer seizures. It is also being studied as an anticancer agent.

8

Improving Your Overall Well-Being

Enjoying the best sex takes more than simply ensuring that you have no major health problems that interfere. It also means taking a look at your lifestyle to be sure your overall well-being supports pleasurable sex. Many herbs can help optimize your health, by giving you more energy, helping you relieve stress, aiding you in overcoming addictions, and assisting you in losing any excess weight. See whether any of these herbs may benefit you *and* your sex life.

Herbs to Increase Your Energy

If you feel fatigued or have a lack of energy, it's no surprise that you may not get too excited about sex. The best way to regain energy is to identify and alleviate whatever is making you feel so fatigued—a health problem, too much stress, side effects from medication, or lack of sleep, for example. These herbs may also help restore your energy levels and restore your sex life as well: *astragalus, fo-ti, ginkgo, ginseng,* and *spirulina.*

Herbs to Reduce Stress

It's almost impossible to avoid stress, but you *can* control your reaction to it. Uncontrolled stress is at the heart of many ills, including impotence and other sex problems. But these herbs can help: *catnip, chamomile, damiana, dong quai, ginseng, gotu kola, guarana, kava,* and *licorice.*

Overcoming Addictions

Often we assume that addictive substances make our sex lives better—that's even why we use them at times. But just the opposite is true. Alcohol, tobacco, and street drugs all impair sexual ability. Herbs can help you deal with overcoming these addictions, allowing you to enjoy sex more than before. Try the following: *barley, cayenne, ginseng, lobelia,* and *spirulina.*

Weight Loss

Extra weight can inhibit your sex life in many ways. It makes movement difficult. It contributes to health problems such as high blood pressure, diabetes, and heart problems that impair sexual function. It makes you feel less attractive. And, the truth is, it may turn off your partner. Herbs can help you achieve weight loss. Take a look at these to see if they are appropriate for you: *cayenne, cinnamon, lobelia, spirulina,* and *wild yam.*

Astragalus

Astragalus membranaceous, a. mongholicus, and others

These perennials are native to Northern Asia and sport hairy stems and black roots.

The basics of astragalus

This family of plants has found use in Chinese medicine for more than two millennia. This herb has a range of specific uses, but is most popular as a general tonic or energizer, especially to combat weakness and fatigue. Animal studies have shown astragalus to be an immune-system builder, especially in the presence of chronic health problems.

Parts used

The root of astragalus is used medicinally.

Chemical content

Astragalus contains polysaccharides and saponins, chemicals that have immune-system-building properties. Other substances are still being identified.

Dosing instructions and availability

Astragalus is available through health food stores and herb shops in the form of capsules, drops, extract, tea, tincture, and fresh and dried root. A common dosage is 1–4 grams of dried root per day. For other forms, follow the product instructions.

Cautions

Reports of side effects are rare. Astragalus is generally considered safe.

Added benefits

This herb touts a long list of possible benefits:
- Anti-inflammatory
- Possible moderation of blood sugar levels
- Inhibition of cancer growth
- Diuretic
- Improved heart function after heart attack
- Anti-viral (destroys the Coxsackie B virus, which attacks the heart)

Barley

Hordeum distichon

Barley grows as a hollow-stemmed grass topped with long bristles that hold the rows of grain.

The basics of barley

Barley has been around for centuries—it was even one of the first crops planted in Virginia in 1611. Barley contains 11 times more calcium than cow's milk, and in years past, was used to dilute cow's milk for infants. It is also one of the first cereals offered to babies.

Barley juice can be an inexpensive, natural way to help you quit smoking, which is a major cause of sex problems such as impotence. Smoking restricts the blood flow through your body, preventing adequate blood flow in the genital areas. This may cause impotence, loss of desire, or simply less sexual pleasure. Using barley to quit smoking helps reverse the damage. Barley cleanses cells and balances the chemicals in your body, which helps to neutralize the toxic effects of nicotine while keeping you feeling in balance. Barley contains a high level of vitamin B_{12}, which helps strengthen and build up your blood. This enables you to fight fatigue and anemia, preserving your strength to fight nicotine cravings.

Parts used

The green (unripe) grass and ripe grain are both used medicinally.

Using Barley to Quit Smoking

Many new prescription and over-the-counter medications can help you quit smoking. However, not everyone is able to use them, because of side effects or even financial concerns. Have you been knocked over by the price of some of the over-the-counter antismoking products? Using juice made from powdered barley can be an easy, inexpensive alternative.

Chemical content

Besides a range of vitamins, barley also contains these active ingredients:
- Beta-glucan, a fiber with cholesterol-lowering benefits
- Chlorophyll
- The mineral calcium

Dosing instructions and availability

Barley is available in grocery stores as a grain, flour, or tea or in food products such as soups. Check health food stores for barley juice, tea, capsules, and powder. For appropriate dosages, consult the product instructions.

Cautions

Barley in all its forms is considered safe. The only known side effect is digestive discomfort in people who can't digest gluten.

Added benefits

- Lowers cholesterol
- May lower blood glucose levels
- Protects against colon cancer

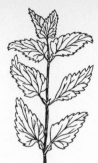

Catnip

Nepeta cataria

Spikes of small white flowers top stems bearing fuzzy, gray-green leaves with serrated edges. Catnip is a perennial that grows throughout the world.

The basics of catnip

The North American Indians used catnip as a sedative to calm nerves and to calm the colic in young children. Because catnip contains chemicals that are similar to sedatives, it may be used to promote better or more restful sleep. Its mild tranquilizing effects also help calm nerves, stress, and anxiety.

Catnip's sedative and relaxing effects may help you quit smoking. Catnip drops have been used by many to curb their cravings for nicotine.

Parts used

Catnip leaves are used.

Chemical content

Nepetalactone is a substance found in the essential oil of catnip that may have sedative properties.

Dosing instructions and availability

You can find catnip drops, capsules, extract, and tincture in health food stores. You may also be able to find catnip as an ingredient in tea. Tea can be made using 2 teaspoons dried catnip per cup of water. Drink 1–3 times per day. For all other forms, follow the instructions on the label.

Cautions

Catnip is generally considered safe.

Added benefits

Have the flu? Catnip can help by reducing your fever. Have a problem with low weight or no or low appetite? Catnip is also known for its ability to stimulate the appetite. Yet another possible benefit of catnip is that it is thought to reduce the risk of cataracts as you age.

Cayenne or Capsicum

Capsicum annuum

Cayenne is a tropical perennial shrub with long, podlike berries.

The basics of cayenne

Spicy food, ornamental pods, criminal deterrent—these are probably the first uses you think of for cayenne pepper. But this tropical perennial shrub with long, podlike berries can also help with symptoms that may inhibit your sex life.

Cayenne made it into European cuisine thanks to Christopher Columbus's trips to the Americas. It has grown for centuries in other areas as well. Cayenne was used by the Greeks, and its formal name, *capsicum,* means "to bite." Ayurvedic medicine, the traditional form of medicine used in India, considers capsicum to be one of the best medicines around. Capsicum is thought to be a strong stimulant and a powerful tool for those who are trying to overcome an addiction to alcohol.

Weight loss may be easier when using capsicum. It promotes perspiration and increases thermogenesis, which is the production of heat in the body.

Parts used

Berries of the cayenne bush are used.

Chemical content

Cayenne has several active ingredients that have helpful benefits:
  • Vitamins A and C

- Capsaicin, a powerful stimulant and anti-inflammatory
- Salicylate, an aspirin-like substance, which works to prevent and treat headaches

Dosing instructions and availability

This herb is as close as your grocery store spice section. You can also find cayenne in pill or extract form at health food stores. Creams containing capsaicin are readily available in drugstores. Or you can make your own liniment by boiling 1 tablespoon of cayenne in 1 pint of cider vinegar. Bottle while still hot.

Cautions

Don't use cayenne if you have intestinal disorders. It can make these conditions worse. Also, prolonged contact with the skin can cause blistering. Keep cayenne out of your eyes (wear rubber gloves when working with it).

Added benefits

Capsicum is also heart-healthy. It cleanses and nourishes the blood vessels, while also strengthening the artery walls. It also discourages the formation of blood clots, which may lead to strokes or heart attacks. Capsicum also helps to lower the amount of cholesterol in the blood stream.

But probably the best-known quality of cayenne is its ability to provide relief from arthritis pain. Capsaicin, which is an ingredient of cayenne, is often used in arthritis cream formulas. It provides heat to the affected area, while also acting as a pain reliever. Cayenne can reduce inflammation of arthritic joints, also lowering the pain. This allows you to move more freely and enjoy sex. Studies show that used externally, capsicum interferes with Substance P, a chemical believed to transmit pain impulses.

Other external and internal uses for the pepper abound:

- Relieving gas and diarrhea
- Easing symptoms of asthma
- Reducing pain of toothaches and sore throats
- Lowering fever

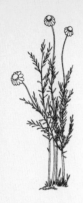

Chamomile

Chamaelum nobile, Matricaria recutita

This annual plant produces fragrant, daisy-like flowers. It is also called German chamomile, and is different than Roman or English chamomile.

The basics of chamomile

Chamomile tea and flowers have been valued for their healing power since early Egyptian times. Strewn on floors to freshen the air, used to cover up the smell and taste of rancid meat, and repelling insects are all early uses of this herb. Chamomile may serve as a mild sedative, helping you to relax when you feel too stressed.

Parts used

The chamomile flower is used.

Chemical content

Chamomile contains these ingredients:

- Alpha-bisabolol, a substance that relaxes muscles and comes from the volatile oil of the chamomile flower
- Flavonoids, which have antispasmodic and anti-inflammatory action
- Chamazolene, and anti-inflammatory and anti-allergy substance
- Polysaccharides, which stimulate the immune system

Dosing instructions and availability

Chamomile tea is available in grocery stores, drugstores, and health food stores. Other forms of chamomile, such as oil, are available from health food stores. The plant is easy to grow. You can collect the flowers, dry them, and make your own tea. Or purchase oil or tea at supermarkets or health food stores. Follow the instructions on the product label. For tea, use 2–3 teaspoons of dried flower per cup of water.

Cautions

Chamomile is generally considered safe. However, if you are allergic to ragweed or chrysanthemums, you may also have an allergic reaction to chamomile.

Added benefits

The many uses of chamomile can be summarized in three categories that cover a lot of individual ills:

- Anti-inflammatory
- Antispasmodic
- Anti-infective

Cinnamon

Cinnamomum zeylanicum

Cinnamon is the name given to several types of evergreens that grow in the West Indies and Asia. The bark has the distinctive reddish-brown color that is associated with this herb.

The basics of cinnamon

Cinnamon has been used in many cultures for relieving stomach and other problems. It has also been suggested as an aid to weight loss, perhaps because the volatile oil stimulates the production of bile, which helps break down fats in the digestive tract.

Parts used

The bark of the cinnamon tree is used. Occasionally the flower is used.

Chemical content

Cinnamon contains an essential oil, which is made up of several chemicals, including eugenol, the same oil found in cloves.

Dosing instructions and availability

Cinnamon can be found in various forms in places ranging from your local supermarket to health food stores and herb shops. You may find it in capsules, oil, drops, powder, tea, and tincture. It is also added to many herbal blends. A common dosage is 2 grams of capsules taken 1–2 times per day. For other forms, follow product instructions. It is recommended that you take cinnamon with food or drink.

Cautions

Cinnamon is generally considered safe. Some people have allergic reactions to cinnamon, especially in the mouth and on the skin. People with ulcers may want to avoid medicinal use of cinnamon, since it stimulates the production of acids. Cinnamon oil should only be used externally. Pregnant women should not use cinnamon medicinally, as it can cause increased heart rate and then slow down the central nervous system.

Added benefits

Cinnamon has many uses:
- Relieves diarrhea and nausea
- Relieves congestion
- Increases blood circulation
- Aids in the digestion process, especially the metabolism of fats
- Fights fungal infection
- Aids in weight loss
- Aids in fighting yeast infections

Damiana

Turnera diffusa

Damiana is a small, shrub-like plant native to Mexico.

The basics of damiana

The history behind damiana begins in Mexico. The story goes that it was an old Mexican folk remedy used to treat various urinary and sexual problems. Even the Maya Indians of Yucatan believed in the healing benefits of damiana. They called it *mizib-coc,* meaning "plant for asthma." Damiana has been used as a general tonic for both men and women, helping to fight fatigue and increase energy. Exactly how it works in the body is yet unknown.

Parts used

The leaves of the damiana shrub are the most commonly used part of the plant. However, it is not unheard of for some herbal preparations to also contain the stem of the shrub.

Chemical content

The damiana shrub contains the following:
- The chemicals arbutin and damianian
- Essential oils
- Resin, a sticky, yellow substance
- Starch
- Sugars
- Tannins

Dosing instructions and availability

Damiana is widely available in health food stores. Many "mainstream" stores, such as discount stores and drugstores, now carry lines of herbal products, often even in generic forms. You may be able to locate damiana there. You can find it as pills or extract or tea.

Even though there are no known side effects from taking damiana, it is generally suggested that you use it for two months, discontinuing usage if no positive effects are noted. Many herbs take at least four to six weeks to be of any benefit, so two months should be enough time to tell if it is helping you have better sex or not! Follow the dosing instructions found on the label. There is no set dosage amount, so if in doubt, start with a lesser amount, and increase if needed.

Cautions

While almost everyone would like to improve their sex life, a little caution is always a good thing. Damiana is not considered to be a very strong or potent herb, and there are really no known side effects. However, because there are also no scientific studies available on damiana, all we know about it comes from personal experience and its use in history.

There is some information that indicates that damiana may interfere with iron absorption. It would be a good idea, if you give damiana a try, to also increase your iron intake. This can be easily accomplished by increasing the iron in your diet. Foods high in iron include: dark green leafy vegetables, eggs, tomato juice, nuts, red meats, and fruits. You may also choose to take extra iron in supplement form. Ask your healthcare provider to check your iron levels if you have any questions.

Possible drug interactions

There is no current information on damiana's having a negative re-action with any other drugs or medications. However, there is some evidence that it may alter sugar levels in the bloodstream, so if you are diabetic or have any other type of problem with regulating your blood sugar levels, consult your healthcare provider before us-ing damiana.

Added benefits

Generally speaking, damiana has long been thought to help a large and quite diverse group of ailments. From its being a laxative to be-ing an aphrodisiac, you would be hard pressed to find a more unique herb available today. Just look at the wide range of physical ailments and conditions that damiana may help:

- Relieves bronchial irritation, possibly providing relief from respiratory conditions such as asthma
- Relieves coughs due to respiratory conditions or even the common cold
- Improves and aids digestion and acts as a laxative by help-ing the muscular contractions of the intestines
- Helps regain strength in limbs
- Alleviates various cold and flu symptoms
- Relieves irritation of urinary mucus membranes, provid-ing relief from urinary conditions
- Increases fertility

Damiana has the reputation of being an aphrodisiac primarily for women, but can be helpful for both men *and* women.

Dong Quai
Angelica sinensis

This perennial has purple stems, clusters of white flowers, and thick, branched roots.

The basics of dong quai

Records as far back as 588 B.C. show dong quai recommended for the treatment of painful menstrual cycles. In both China and Japan, dong quai has long held a reputation as "women's ginseng" and is second in sales only to licorice root.

Even though dong quai is best known for its female healing properties, it may act like a sedative for men.

Parts used

Dong quai roots are used.

Chemical content

Dong quai contains several known ingredients, some of which can be harmful when used in purified forms. Ingredients include the following:

- Phytoestrogens, which act like estrogen in a woman's body
- Psoralen, bergapten, and other coumarin derivatives, which dilate blood vessels and relax muscles
- Safrole, a substance found in the essential oil, which in pure form can cause cancer

Dosing instructions and availability

This herb is available in herb shops and health food stores. Dong quai comes in capsule, extract, powder, and other forms. It is also included in some beverages marketed to enhance sexual pleasure. Often, it is an ingredient in Chinese soups. When taking the capsule, extract, powder, or other medicinal forms, follow instructions on the product's label. A common dose is 3–5 grams per day. Avoid purified forms of dong quai.

Cautions

Dong quai can cause miscarriage. Coumarin derivatives may cause sun sensitivity and cancer. Purified safrole can cause cancer.

Added benefits

Dong quai also has antibiotic qualities, quite possibly being able to keep you from getting sick. It is a blood builder, which helps to heal all wounds and treat those who suffer from anemia. It is a bowel lubricant, helping those who suffer from constipation. Other benefits of dong quai include the following:

- Enhances vitamin E activity in those who are deficient
- Relieves insomnia
- Nourishes the brain
- Relieves arthritis pain
- Acts as an expectorant to treat bronchial conditions or coughs
- Helps to relieve gas and indigestion
- By increasing estrogen levels, dong quai may be used in the treatment of infertility
- May stimulate the appetite

Fo-ti or He Shou Wu

Polygonum multiflorum

This perennial evergreen vine is one of the main herbs used in Chinese medicine. It is also called knotweed.

The basics of fo-ti

Fo-ti supposedly got its Chinese name from a man who used the herb and became sexually active after being impotent. It is also used for a general stimulant and tonic, having anti-aging properties.

Parts used

The root of the fo-ti vine is used.

Chemical content

Fo-ti contains the following substances:

- Anthraquinone substances—emodine and rhein—that stimulate the bowels
- Lecithin, a fatty substance that may help lower cholesterol

Dosing instructions and availability

This herb can be found in herb shops or health food stores. It comes in the form of powder, pill, or extract. It is also added to some beverages. Follow the label instructions on the product or contact an herbalist.

Cautions

Few side effects have been noted with fo-ti. However, limit its use so that your body does not become dependent on its laxative effects.

Added benefits

Other uses of fo-ti include the following:

- Diuretic
- Cholesterol reducer
- Aid to digestion
- Support of the endocrine system
- Anti-aging properties

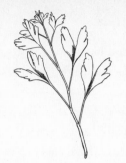

Ginkgo
Ginkgo biloba

This deciduous ornamental tree, native to China, has fan-shaped leaves and yellow seeds that give off a rather unpleasant odor.

The basics of ginkgo

Ginkgo is at times referred to as the "smart herb," because of its ability to enhance the memory and even possibly slow down the progression of Alzheimer's disease. Ginkgo doesn't perform miracles, but does this by increasing the blood flow throughout the body, enabling the user to feel stronger and more alert. By stimulating and improving blood circulation throughout the body, ginkgo provides more oxygen to the brain, heart, and all other body parts, including those required for sex. This results in your feeling more energetic, even during times when you are also under stress.

Parts used

The leaves and nuts of the ginkgo tree are used.

Chemical content

- Gingko extract contains the active ingredients of flavone glycosides and terpenes
- Gingkolides are steroidal substances in the tree currently under research

Dosing instructions and availability

This herb is available in grocery, drug, and health food stores, as well as through herb shops and mail order companies. It comes in pills, extract, and added to products.

Follow the instructions on the product's label. It takes several months to begin to feel the effects of ginkgo. Many herbal practitioners believe that the amount of the active ingredients in ginkgo leaves are too diluted. To get enough ginkgo to be of much benefit, it is suggested that you take ginkgo in a standardized form, such as an extract or capsule. The usual dosing amount is 40 mg of extract 3 times per day or 60 to 240 mg in capsule form per day. Take this herb with meals to avoid stomach upset.

Cautions

Don't use more than 240 mg of ginkgo per day. Ginkgo can act as a blood thinner, so if you are already taking blood-thinning medication (including aspirin), avoid this herb. There have been reports of diarrhea, restlessness, and irritability when using ginkgo.

Added benefits

Take a look at what ginkgo may do for you:
- Lowers blood pressure
- Helps to prevent blood clots from forming, possibly preventing heart attack or stroke
- Improves mental ability, such as memory, clarity, and alertness
- May slow down the advancement of Alzheimer's disease
- Alleviates depression
- Provides relief from tinnitis, or ringing in the ears
- Relieves muscle aches and pains
- Relieves impotence

Add to this list anti-aging. By improving mental functions, helping blood circulation, and being an antioxidant, ginkgo may help you live a longer, healthier, fuller life.

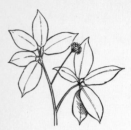

Ginseng

Panax ginseng, p. quinquefolius

A low-growing, shade-loving plant, ginseng produces red berries on stems surrounded by clusters of five leaves. The plant grows slowly, taking from two to five years for the root to be ready for harvest.

The basics of ginseng

Ginseng is an extremely expensive but wonderful herb that has been used medicinally for thousands of years. Its botanical name, *panax,* comes from a Greek word, *panacea,* which means "all healing." In China, it is sometimes referred to as the man's plant, referring to the shape of the ginseng root. Ginseng roots are considered to be more valuable because of their increased effectiveness as they age. Ginseng is sometimes referred to as the herbal "Fountain of Youth."

Despite its widespread use, no one is sure yet how ginseng works. There have been studies done by Russian scientists that have shown that ginseng stimulates physical and mental activities and improves endocrine gland functions, while having a positive effect on the sex glands. Women and men have reported greater sexual pleasure from the use of ginseng. This may be due to its energy-increasing properties as well as its effects on the endocrine glands. Ginseng's energizing effects help fight fatigue and stress and can even aid in breaking addictions.

Parts used

The root of the ginseng plant is used.

Chemical content

Ginseng contains ginsenosides, steroidal substances that affect the central nervous system and help the body adapt to environmental and mental stress.

Dosing instructions and availability

This herb is easily available in powder, pill, and extract form at your grocery store, health food store, drugstore, or herb shop. You can also find ginseng added to many other food products and beverages that are marketed as increasing energy. Common doses are 1–2 grams of root per day or 250 to 1,000 mg of capsules. Amounts of ginseng vary considerably from product to product, so read labels and follow product instructions carefully. (See page 84 for information on the three types of ginseng.)

Cautions

Since ginseng is overharvested and expensive, some unscrupulous manufacturers substitute ingredients. Purchase products that guarantee their contents or buy ground ginseng root to avoid possible side effects from unknown substances.

Side effects from ginseng are rare, but include nervousness and diarrhea. Those suffering from hypoglycemia, diabetes, low or high blood pressure, or any heart disorder should closely monitor their symptoms when using ginseng. Also, women should not use ginseng in large amounts, or for too long, as it increases testosterone production, which is a male sex hormone, and may result in a lowering of the voice and increase of body or facial hair.

Possible drug interactions

Ginseng may also interact with certain types of medications, both over-the-counter and prescription. More specifically, some antibiotic, tranquilizer, sedative, and antihistamine medications may interact with ginseng, so always use with caution and read all labels.

Added benefits

There is a long, long list of other benefits that you may gain from the use of ginseng. There have been reports of some athletes using ginseng to enhance their athletic performance, while also increasing their endurance. Many athletes also use it for over-all body strengthening and conditioning as well. Others include:

- Improves brain functions, such as memory, clarity, or alertness
- Helps heal the prostate gland
- Aids in the digestive process
- Regulates blood sugar
- Strengthens and stimulates the adrenal glands and reproductive organs
- Stimulates appetite
- May help treat infertility
- Increases mental alertness
- Helps to lower blood pressure
- Helps to prevent heart disease
- Helps to condition the lungs, aiding in the treatment of emphysema, asthma, or chronic bronchitis

Gotu Kola

Centella asiatica

Gotu kola is a small, low-growing perennial plant with small fan-shaped leaves, clusters of small flowers, and small berries. This herb grows pretty much world-wide in tropical areas. It is native to Africa, India, Sri Lanka, and Malaysia. Gotu kola doesn't like cold weather, and can't survive temperatures lower than 30°F.

The basics of gotu kola

For centuries, gotu kola has been used in India to increase one's mental power—including better concentration and improved memory. It has also been widely used in India for longevity. Gotu kola fights fatigue, depression, and anxiety, giving you more energy and desire for sex.

Parts used

Nuts, roots, and seeds of gotu kola are used.

Chemical content

Gotu kola contains the following substances:
- Asiaticoside, one of the active ingredients, which may also be cancer-causing
- The chemicals catechol and epicatechol
- Magnesium, a mineral
- Theobromine, a stimulant similar to caffeine
- Vitamin K

Dosing instructions and availability

Gotu kola is available in extract, drop, dried leaves, and tincture forms at health food stores and herb shops. Common doses are ½–1 dropperful of tincture or drops 2–3 times per day or 2–4 grams of the leaves per day. If using it externally, simply put a few drops of gotu kola extract on a cotton ball, and apply to the affected area.

Cautions

The most commonly cited problem with gotu kola is skin irritation when used externally. Otherwise, it is generally considered safe. However, some evidence in animals indicates that gotu kola when used repeatedly may cause cancer.

Added benefits

Gotu kola is used in the treatment of burns, since it can stimulate tissue growth by increasing the production of collagen. In clinical trials in Brazil and other countries, gotu kola has been successfully used to treat all kinds of skin conditions. These include surgical wounds, gangrene, skin grafts, and skin ulcers.

Other uses of gotu kola include the following:
- Shrinks tissues
- Stimulates central nervous system, good for nervous disorders
- Improves heart and liver functions
- Helps eliminate kidney stones
- Aids in elimination of excess fluids
- Strengthens connective tissues
- Increases energy and endurance
- Heals tissues by stimulating the growth of collagen
- Acts as a blood purifier

Guarana

Paullinia cupana and p. sorbilis

Guarana (pronounced guar-an-A) is a climbing evergreen shrub with yellow-orange fruits. It is native to South America.

The basics of guarana

Folks in Brazil have long thought guarana to be an aphrodisiac. They make tea and sodas out of guarana seeds, drinking it to get the herb's aphrodisiac effects. Guarana's powers of stimulation may help combat fatigue and stress, helping you feel more energetic, even when it comes to sex.

Parts used

Seeds of the guarana plant are ground into a paste that is then dried.

Chemical content

- Guaranine, which is similar to caffeine
- Tannins, which reduce intestinal inflammation
- Essential oils estragole and anethole

Dosing instructions and availability

Guarana comes as a dried herb or in pill, extract, syrup, or tea form. It may also be found in beverages. Check at health food stores or at markets that sell South American spices. Try 500–1,000 mg of dried guarana or 0.5 to 4 grams of powdered guarana a day. Mix it into boiling water to make a tea, or add it to any soft drink. Follow labeling instructions.

Cautions

Guarana has the same effects as any caffeinated product, so use in moderation. Guarana colas may increase tooth decay.

Added benefits

- General stimulant and tonic
- Reduces fever
- Relieves headaches, including migraines

Hops

Humulus lupulus

This herb is a perennial vine with leaves grouped in three, tiny flowers, and pale green fruit. It is native to North American and Europe.

The basics of hops

You're probably familiar with hops as an ingredient in beer, which gives it a bitter, distinctive flavor. However, hops has been used as a sedative by American Indians for at least a few centuries. Its sedative effects can help promote sleep when you're feeling restless and overstressed. And, interestingly, the older hops gets, the more concentrated are its sedative ingredients.

Parts used

The fruit of hops is used.

Chemical content

Hops contains the following:
- Dimethyl carbinol, a sedative
- Bitter acids, which may promote digestion and fight bacteria and fungi

Dosing instructions and availability

Hops is available through health food stores and herb shops as drops, dried and fresh fruit, and extract. A common dose is 1–2 droppersful of drops.

Cautions

Hops is generally considered safe. But remember not to mix hops with alcohol or any other sedative.

Added benefits

Hops is used for other medicinal purposes as well:
- Reducing restlessness and anxiety
- Aiding digestion
- Killing certain bacteria and fungi
- Destroying some tumor cells

Hydrangea

Hydrangea aborescens

A shrub growing to ten feet tall, hydrangea has woody stems with large, round leaves. Hydrangea produces clusters of white flowers. Note that this hydrangea is native to North America. It is not the same as those usually used as ornamentals. Nor is it the same hydrangea used in traditional Chinese medicine.

The basics of hydrangea

The name hydrangea was derived from a Greek word meaning "water-vessel." Hydrangea was once used by the Cherokee Indians as a diuretic and in the treatment of "calculi," that is, stones or deposits in the kidneys. It is still thought to be an excellent herb to purge the kidneys, as well as an overall tonic. Hydrangea's role as a diuretic may help aid weight loss.

Part used

Only the roots of the hydrangea plant should be used.

Chemical content

Hydrangea contains these substances:
- Essential oils
- Saponin, a soapy substance
- Resin, a yellow, sticky substance

Dosing instructions and availability

This herb is available in pill and extract form from health food stores and herb shops. Follow the product label instructions.

Cautions

Do not use the leaves or buds. Hydrangea root may cause vertigo (dizziness) in some people.

Added benefits

Hydrangea also has the following uses:
- Helps correct bedwetting in children
- Helps treat obesity
- Acts as a laxative
- May relieve urinary tract problems

Juniper
Juniperus communis

Juniper is an evergreen shrub or tree with tightly packed needles, small yellow flowers, and midnight blue berries or cones. This herb produces a distinctive aroma.

The basics of juniper

Juniper's long-standing reputation as a diuretic actually led to the creation of the alcoholic drink gin: In the 1500s a Dutch pharmacist soaked juniper berries in alcohol to make a diuretic potion. Juniper's diuretic properties are probably what has led folks over the centuries to use this herb as a weight-loss aid. It rids the body of fluid by irritating the kidneys and urinary tract.

Parts used

Juniper berries are steamed to release the volatile oil.

Chemical contents

Juniper contains the following substances:

- Terpinen-4-ol, a volatile oil responsible for the berry's diuretic properties, and which may also have anti-inflammatory properties
- Juniperin, a bitter chemical that may help stimulate digestion

Dosing instructions and availability

Juniper berries, extract, oil, syrup, and tincture are available at health food stores and herb shops. A common dosage is 1 tablespoon of syrup taken in the morning and evening.

Cautions

Juniper berries can over-irritate the kidneys and urinary tract, damaging them permanently. To avoid this and other side effects such as diarrhea and convulsions, do not use juniper for more than six weeks at a time. Do not use juniper when taking other diuretic medications. *Pregnant women should avoid juniper, since it can cause miscarriage.*

Added benefits

Juniper is also used for other purposes:
- For relief of menstrual bloating
- For relief of heart failure and high blood pressure
- To treat respiratory problems
- To relieve nerve pain
- To flavor foods and add fragrance to cosmetics

Kava or Kava Kava

Piper methysticum

Kava is a large flowering shrub and a member of the pepper family of plants. The shrub produces knotty roots. It grows only in tropical forests, but its use in nontropical areas is booming.

The basics of kava

Many years ago, kava was "discovered" by the explorer Captain James Cook, who dubbed this herb "intoxicating pepper." Before Cook's discovery, however, the ancient Tahitians and other Pacific Islanders used—and continue to use—kava as a general all-around feel-good tonic and a stimulant.

Kava is also considered to be one of the most powerful herbal muscle relaxants available today. In addition, it is good for calming nerves, fighting anxiety, and alleviating stress. Kava can also help put an insomniac to sleep, while enabling the user to obtain a more restful sleep.

Parts used

The kava root is used.

Chemical content

Kava contains two chemicals that are known to relieve pain: the kavalactones dihydrokavain and dihydromethysticin.

Dosing instructions and availability

Kava can be found in capsule, extract, powder, and root. It's best to use kava that has been prepared by a reputable supplements company, so that the active ingredients will be at a consistent level. Follow labeling instructions carefully.

Cautions

Kava is generally considered to be a safe and mild tranquilizer and an all-around tonic when used in small amounts (up to 250 mg of kavalactones daily). However, if you are already using a medication that has similar effects as kava, be careful! A few cases have been reported of people falling into a coma after combining kava with alcohol or antidepressant or antianxiety medications. Work with your doctor if you want to try kava in addition to or in place of these medications.

In addition, there is some evidence that kava may become addictive. Continuous use can lead to skin and blood problems. Avoid kava when you need to remain alert, such as for driving and operating machinery.

Added benefits

Kava is known to be a good source of pain relief for those suffering from rheumatism. Kava may be used both externally and internally to treat all types of pain. It also serves as a muscle relaxant. All these effects of kava can help you remain pain-free, which can certainly help you enjoy sex more.

Kava's diuretic properties can also help relieve bladder problems.

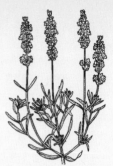

Lavender
Lavendula angustifolia

This evergreen shrubby herb produces long spikes with pebbly, gray-green leaves and small purple flowers. The herb has a distinctive, pleasant aroma.

The basics of lavender

This herb originated in the Mediterranean areas, but quickly found its way to the rest of the world. For centuries, lavender has been used as a general tonic to relieve stress, calm nerves, and promote sleep, among other uses. It accomplishes this through its sedative and antispasmodic qualities, due to its volatile oil and the fragrance released by the oil. How the oil works on the body, however, has yet to be determined, though studies have shown lavender aromatherapy and tea to be effective aids to relieving stress and promoting sleep.

Parts used

The flowers and oil from the lavender plant are used.

Chemical contents

Lavender contains a volatile oil made up of many other components that have yet to be identified. Tannins in lavender contribute to its external use as a wound healer.

Dosing instructions and availability

Lavender is available at supermarkets, drugstores, health food stores, and herb shops. You can find it in many forms: dried flowers, oil, tincture, extract, and others. You can also find it added to bath products. A common dosage for tea is 1–2 teaspoons flowers per cup of water taken several times per day. Externally, 1–5 drops of oil in bathwater is a common dosage.

Cautions

Lavender is generally considered safe when used in recommended dosages. Large dosages taken internally can cause too much sedation and externally can cause skin reactions.

Added benefits

Lavender is used for other purposes as well:
- Relieving digestive problems
- Treating wounds
- Strengthening the nervous system
- Relieving discomfort after childbirth
- Possibly regulating blood sugar levels, as indicated in animal studies

Licorice

Glycyrrhiza glabra

Licorice is a shrub with spreading roots and rhizomes. It is native to subtropical areas, including Southeast Europe and Southwest Asia.

The basics of licorice

Licorice has a long history of medicinal use, dating from the Greeks, who used licorice for various respiratory illnesses, including asthma and coughs. Currently, licorice is still often found as an ingredient in cough lozenges.

Alexander the Great also found good uses for licorice. His troops were sent out with a supply of licorice, among their other battle gear. The purpose? Troops were to chew their licorice sticks to alleviate their thirst, while also increasing their energy levels. Licorice is still used as a general tonic and stimulant, to increase your energy. It has been recommended even for people with chronic fatigue syndrome. How it accomplishes its energizing effects on the body, however, is still unknown.

Parts used

The root of the licorice plant is used.

Chemical content

Licorice contains these substances:
- Asparagine and choline, two amino acids
- Fat
- Glycyrretenic acid, a cough suppressant

- Glycyrrhizin and liquiritin, steroidal substances with antibacterial and anti-inflammatory properties
- Gum
- Inositol, a type of alcohol
- Lecithin
- The minerals manganese and phosphorus
- Pentacyclic terpene, a solvent-like substance found in the essential oil
- Proteins
- Sugars
- Vitamins B_1, B_2, B_3, B_6, and E

Dosing instructions and availability

This herb is added to many candies found in grocery stores. You can also find the herb and teas containing it in health food stores and herb shops. Other products containing licorice may be found in drugstores.

Eat licorice sticks or foods prepared with licorice as an ingredient. For teas and other forms of licorice, follow product instructions. Common doses are 1–2 grams powdered root, 2–4 ml liquid extract, or 250–500 mg solid extract, each taken 3 times per day.

Cautions

If you are pregnant; have diabetes, glaucoma, heart disease, high blood pressure, or severe menstrual problems; or if you have suffered a stroke, you should not use licorice without first consulting your healthcare provider.

Even if you do not suffer from the above illnesses, you should not use licorice for more than 4–6 weeks at a time. Licorice has the potential to cause high blood pressure, swelling, high sodium levels, and low potassium levels.

Added benefits

Licorice has many other positive effects on the human body. For example, licorice contains glycyrrhizin, which kills bacteria, making licorice a wonderful tooth decay preventative. Here are other uses for licorice:

- Stimulates the production of interferon, which may be helpful to those with immune disorders
- Cleanses the colon
- Decreases muscular spasms
- Helps adrenal gland function
- Relieves respiratory diseases, such as asthma and emphysema
- Fights fever
- Helps fight hypoglycemia by raising blood sugar levels to normal levels
- Helps fight arthritis
- Normalizes ovulation and relieves symptoms of PMS and menopause
- Fights sore throats

Lobelia

Lobelia inflata

This short annual plant with clusters of almost-purple leaves and delicate violet-blue flowers doesn't appear to be the tough fighter that it is. Lobelia may help overcome many addictions, especially nicotine and food.

The basics of lobelia

Another common name for lobelia is "Indian tobacco," probably because the active substance in lobelia creates a similar response in your body as the nicotine found in cigarettes. Stopping smoking and losing weight both have direct benefits for your sex life. Lobelia may help with either concern. Your body's response to lobelia may greatly reduce nicotine cravings. Lobeline also even makes smoking cigarettes taste bad—soon you may find yourself not even want to smoke. And just as people believe that nicotine suppresses the appetite, lobelia, too, has similar effects.

This relaxant promotes sleep or even more restful sleep. Lobelia relaxes the bronchial muscles, helping those suffering from bronchitis or even asthma to breathe easier. It even works as a cough suppressant when you have a cold, as well as a fever reducer when you have the flu.

Parts used

Lobelia flowers, seeds, and leaves are used.

Chemical content

Lobelia contains lobeline, which acts somewhat like nicotine in your body, relaxing the smooth muscles.

Dosing instructions and availability

This herb is available in herb shops and health food stores. It can be found as capsule, dried herb, extract, and powder. Antismoking aids containing lobelia, such as gum, cannot be sold in the United States because levels of active ingredient vary greatly from product to product. Follow the label instructions carefully and consult an herbalist.

When using lobelia, increase your amount of water that you drink to help flush the nicotine and other toxins from your body.

Cautions

The U.S. FDA considers lobelia to be poisonous. Lobelia can cause serious side effects such as nausea and vomiting even when used at recommended doses. A dose of lobelia higher than 50 mg has the potential to suppress breathing and depress your blood pressure, possibly leading to coma.

Added benefits

Lobelia is a muscle relaxant and has even been used during childbirth to help the process and keep the mother relaxed. This relaxant promotes sleep or even more restful sleep. Lobelia relaxes the bronchial muscles, helping those suffering from bronchitis or even asthma to breathe more easily.

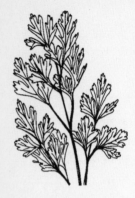

Parsley

Petroselinum crispum, p. sativum, p. hortense

Besides its use as a garnish for fancy meals or for cooking, the bright green, compact, leafy parsley plant can also be helpful to your sex drive. Chinese parsley (cilantro) is not related to this common parsley.

The basics of parsley

In folk history, parsley was used for many female problems, as well as a range of other uses. Women used it to increase milk production when nursing and to facilitate childbirth, as well as to increase their libido. Its diuretic effects have caused parsley to be used as an aid to weight loss, as well.

Parts used

Leaves and stems of parsley are used. For medicinal purposes, an oil is made from the seeds.

Chemical content

The following substances can be found in parsley:
- Apiin, a sticky, aromatic camphor
- Apiol and myristicin, which stimulate the uterus and reduce fever and are acids found in the essential oil
- The minerals calcium, iodine, iron, phosphorus, and potassium
- Mucilage, a plant gum

- Myristicene, a fatty acid
- Pinene, similar to turpentine
- Vitamins A, B-complex, and C
- Chlorophyll, a breath freshener
- Other chemicals, including bergapten, furanocumarin, isoimperatorin, and petroselinic acid.

Dosing instructions and availability

Parsley is available fresh or dried at any supermarket. It is also easy to grow. Seeds or plants are available through most plant nurseries. Oil and root extract are available through health food stores. For medicinal purposes, place 1–2 teaspoons of dried leaves, root, or seeds in 1 cup of hot water (not boiling water—too much heat destroys the delicate oil).

Cautions

Large amounts of parsley oil could stimulate contractions in pregnant women. Long-term use of the oil can cause digestive irritation and other adverse reactions. Parsley oil can also worsen kidney problems.

Added benefits

Other uses of parsley include:
- Possible prevention of the spread of cancer cells
- Relief of gas, while stimulating the digestive system to function properly
- Freshening breath
- Diuretic
- Fever reduction

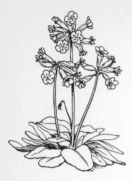

Primrose or Cowslip
Primula veris

This cool-loving plant grows 4 to 8 inches high and produces clusters of bright green leaves with yellow, fragrant flowers in early spring.

The basics of primrose

This herb has been used for centuries in Europe as a mild sedative and for respiratory problems. Although little is known about how this herb works, primrose has also traditionally been used as an aid to weight loss.

Parts used

Dried roots and rhizomes and flowers are used medicinally.

Chemical content

Primrose contains many substances, including the following:
- Gamma-linolenic acid (GLA) and linoleic acid, which may be helpful for maintaining heart health
- Tannins, astringents used for healing skin problems
- Saponins, substances in the roots that may help lower blood pressure and have anti-inflammatory and anti-pain properties
- Flavonoids, which have antispasmodic and anti-inflammatory properties

Dosing instructions and availability

Primrose is available in many health food stores. It takes the form of dried flowers, extract, syrup, and tincture and can be found in herbal teas and cough preparations. A common dosage is 1–2 ml extract up to 3 times per day. Follow product instructions for proper dosage.

Cautions

Not much is known about the safety of primrose. Some people notice stomach problems and nausea after using the root. Others have noted skin irritation when handling primrose flowers.

Added benefits

Primrose is an excellent source of unsaturated fats, which may help reduce blood pressure while alleviating any skin disorders that you may have. Other benefits from taking primrose include:
- Reduces blood pressure
- A good remedy for laryngitis, bronchitis, colds, and coughs
- Alleviates skin conditions including eczema and skin dryness
- Used to treat alcoholism
- Used in the treatment of colitis
- May relieve the pain and stiffness of arthritis
- May relieve symptoms of menopause and PMS

Sarsaparilla
Smilax officinalis

Sarsaparilla is a prickly, climbing, perennial vine with long, creeping roots. Sometimes it is referred to as Chinese root. Sarsaparilla is native to the Caribbean.

The basics of sarsparilla

The most common American use of sarsparilla was as an ingredient of a soft drink similar to root beer. Medicinally, it was used by American Indian women as a tea drunk after childbirth to help expel the placenta. It is thought that the Crees used sarsaparilla in the treatment of syphilis.

Sarsaparilla contains a testosterone-like substance that may be what causes it to increase your energy level. This may explain its long-time use as an energy builder, fighting fatigue and stress.

Parts used

The rhizome (roots) of sarsaparilla is used.

Chemical content

Sarsaparilla contains these ingredients:
- The minerals copper, iron, manganese, sodium, sulfur, and zinc
- Essential oils
- Fatty acids, including sitosterol and stigmasterin
- Glycosides, derivatives of sugars
- Resin, an amber-colored sticky substance

- Saponins, sarsapogenin, and smilagenin, steroidal substances
- Sugars
- Vitamins A and D
- The chemical parillin

Dosing instructions and availability

This herb is available in some beverages found primarily at health food stores. You may also find it as an extract or tincture. A common dose is ¼–½ teaspoon of the tincture 1 to 3 times per day. Follow the product label instructions.

Cautions

Sarsparilla is considered safe. However, doses greater than recommended amounts can cause stomach upset.

Added benefits

Other uses of this plant includes the following:
- Protects from radiation exposure
- Regulates hormone levels
- Acts as a diuretic
- Lowers blood pressure
- Helps clear up skin conditions, such as psoriasis, shingles, and eczema
- Acts as a laxative
- Relieves symptoms of inflammatory diseases like arthritis

Spirulina

Algae pratenis

This is a blue-green algae that grows in freshwater lakes.

The basics of spirulina

For centuries, this algae has been used for food and medicinal purposes in many places throughout the world. Although it grows among scum and bacteria, spirulina is one of the most naturally sterile foods found in nature. Here's what spirulina has done for others.

By boosting your energy level and increasing your overall health, spirulina helps you enjoy all aspects of the sexual experience more—even if you're relatively healthy to begin with. It may help you lose weight by satisfying hunger, though no studies have proven this claim. It keeps you healthier by aiding the absorption of minerals.

Need to quit smoking? Stop drinking? End a chemical dependency? Spirulina can help you in those areas, too, by feeding the body and brain and keeping it healthy, while removing toxins from the body.

Parts used

The entire spirulina plant is used.

Chemical content

Spirulina provides over 25 times more calcium than cow's milk, as well as iron. Spirulina is considered to be the highest source in the world of beta-carotene, vitamin B_{12}, and gamma linoleic acid (GLA). Add in all nine essential amino acids and most of the nonessential amino acids, and you have an amazingly healthy, energizing food supplement.

Dosing instructions and availability

You can find this algae in most health food stores in capsule and powder forms and in herbal blends. Follow the label instructions carefully.

Cautions

Spirulina can contain high levels of mercury and other contaminants. Use a reliable source.

Added benefits

For starters, spirulina has the ability to build stronger blood, cells, and tissues, shortening healing time after an injury or illness. At the same time, spirulina protects the heart, lowers cholesterol, and balances your blood sugar levels. Spirulina also is a memory and brain enhancer by providing your brain with vital nutrients.

Valerian

Valeriana officinalis

This herb sports tall stems with rich, dark-green leaves and light-colored flowers.

The basics about valerian

Another name valerian is known by is all-heal. This is a description of valerian's reputation as an antidote for just about everything. Ancient Romans used valerian to treat heart conditions, primarily heart arrhythmias and palpitations. Valerian is thought to increase the blood flow and circulation and create a mild sedative and tranquilizing effect. These actions may help give you more energy and relieve stress. However, no one as yet has been able to establish how valerian accomplishes these effects.

Parts used

Roots and rhizomes of valerian are used.

Chemical content

Valerian contains the following:
- Acetic, butyric, and formic acids
- Camphene
- Chatinine
- Essential oils
- Glycosides
- Magnesium
- Pinene

- Valeric acid
- Valerine

Dosing instructions and availability

Valerian is available at health food stores in extract and capsule forms. Because it has the reputation of smelling like "dirty gym socks" and pretty much tastes like you would expect these dirty socks to taste, you may prefer to take this herb by capsule form. A common dose is three 456 mg capsules taken 3 times per day.

Cautions

Valerian is generally considered safe. Because of its sedative effects, avoid taking this herb when driving or operating machinery.

Added benefits

Valerian is sometimes called an "herbal tranquilizer." And no wonder: it has sedative and tranquilizing powers, plus is considered to be one of the best sleep aids around! In the United Kingdom, over 80 sleep aids that are available without a prescription contain valerian as the active ingredient. And better yet, valerian is not considered to be habit-forming and doesn't leave you feeling groggy and sleepy in the morning. But there are many other potential benefits to using valerian, too:

- Improves blood circulation throughout the body
- Reduces mucus and helps treat colds and allergies
- Reduces high blood pressure
- Relieves muscle cramps
- Alleviates the pain of ulcers
- Relieves tension
- Relieves irritable bowels

Wild Yam

Dioscorea villosa

Wild yam is a perennial vine with heart-shaped leaves, green flowers, and potato-like tubers. This herb is native to North America.

The basics of wild yam

American Indians used to consume wild yams to relieve a variety of aches and pains, including labor pains during the childbirth process. This herb was also used by American slaves.

Wild yam's estrogen-like substances and other hormonal-like substances may aid weight loss. However, as yet there are no formal studies supporting the effectiveness of wild yam.

Parts used

The rhizomes and roots of wild yam are used.

Chemical content

Wild yam contains a naturally occurring plant steroid, called dioxgenin, which is a natural precursor to progesterone (one of the female hormones). Other ingredients include:

- Alkaloids, bitter substances that occur in seed plants
- The chemicals kioscin and steroidal saponins
- Phytosterols, fatty substances found in plants
- Starch
- Tannins

Dosing instructions and availability

Wild yam cream is available at health food stores and drugstores in the form of capsules, cream, drops, extract, powder, and tincture. A common dosage for internal use is tincture ½ teaspoon twice a day, two 505 mg capsules daily, or 2–4 ml liquid extract daily. For external creams, follow product instructions. Some prescription creams also contain wild yam—follow the prescription instructions.

For best absorption, wild yam creams should also be applied to the thinner skin of the body, such as the chest, breasts, lower abdomen, inner thighs, inner arms, wrist, and neck. It can be applied in the vaginal area to alleviate vaginal itching and dryness.

Cautions

Wild yam is generally considered safe. However, because it may influence hormones, pregnant women and anyone undergoing hormone therapy should avoid this herb.

When using wild yam as an external cream, keep in mind that the skin you are rubbing it on may become sensitive to it. You should rotate the areas you apply it to.

Added benefits

Some other benefits of using wild yam include:
- Alleviates kidney stones
- Relieves gallbladder disorders by promoting the production of bile
- Helps to regulate blood sugar levels, alleviating hypoglycemia
- Relieves pain associated with arthritis

9

Sex Herb Combinations

Take a step into your local supermarket, discount store, drugstore, health food store, ethnic foods store, herb shop—even into your local convenience store—or "surf" into one of the many online shopping areas of the Internet. You'll probably be astonished to see that herbs are available *everywhere* these days, and in every form imaginable! First look in their medicine area; you'll find boxes, bottles, and bags, all full of herbal products. Then look in the candy section; there you'll see herbs as ingredients in "sports bars" or "energy bars." Next, take a stroll to the beverage section; look for an array of colorful bottles bearing names like "SoBe," "Arizona Tea," or "Hansen's." You'll also notice a wall of boxes containing a range of herbal teas.

Given this wealth of herbal products, what exactly should you buy? You may have a clear idea of which herbs you wish to try. In that case, simply find the individual herbal products in the form you desire—with guaranteed ingredients—at the best price. But if selecting and using herbs to enhance your sex life seems overwhelming, you may want to take a look at the various herbal combinations now available. These blends of herbs come in a variety of forms: capsule or pill, extract, or even beverage or tea.

If you wish to try an herb blend, be sure to read the list of ingredients to make sure the product contains the herbs you wish, in quantities that are appropriate. You'll want to refer to the herbs described in this book, and possibly even consult a knowledgeable store employee or an herbalist or nutritionist about specific brands. The U.S. Food and Drug Administration (FDA) does not allow herbal products to make direct claims about the uses or benefits of the product; however, some products have "sexy" names that imply their intended benefits. Other products have more ho-hum names but contain similar combinations of herbs. In this chapter we'll describe the range of combination herb products available, give examples, and describe the most likely sources for these products.

Capsules, Pills, and Extracts

The products that contain the greatest amount of herbs are the ones found in capsule, pill, or extract form. These herbal blends are sold practically everywhere these days, and under many brand names. Some you'll readily recognize like Centrum or One-A-Day. Others are maybe less recognizable, but also are from reputable manufacturers like Twin Labs or Nature's Pride.

Large stores or nutritional supplement chain stores often sell their own "house" or "generic" brands. If you look at these products closely, though, you may find that in fact they are actually produced by the same well-known manufacturers as the name-brand products. Some products may not have the actual manufacturer listed, but instead may list a telephone number. By calling, you may

Herb blends and other herbal products are easily purchased over the Internet. Here are just a few examples of sites that offer herbs:

- www.gil.net/~maria/herbal.html (Bennett Herbal Products)
- www.maine.com/herbs/ (Quantum Herbal Products)
- www.herbal elements.com/english/ (Herbal Elements)
- www. immuvit.com (American Herbal Products)

be able to find out the actual manufacturer, or at least get more information about the product. Some stores that specialize in herbs and supplements often provide written information about the products.

There are literally hundreds of brands of herb blends available in capsule, pill, extract, juice, and essential oil form. Here are some that we were able to identify. Check your local health food store or herb shop for even more.

Yohimbe-Plus by Irwin Naturals The product guarantees potency level and claims to be the highest potency available currently. The label lists the following sex herbs in these amounts:
- Yohimbe bark powder, 2000 mg
- Licorice root extract, 225 mg
- Damiana, 225 mg
- Saw palmetto, 225 mg
- Siberian ginseng, 225 mg

Please note that the above amounts are for three tablets, which the directions say is the daily dosage amount.

X-A by Nature's Sunshine This company has been in operation—according to the label—since 1972. This bottle doesn't look as flashy or exciting as many others, nor does it glaringly say what it is really intended to do. However, it is marketed as a "glandular system support" dietary supplement. Sex herbs in this supplement include the following:

- Siberian ginseng root
- Saw palmetto berries
- Gotu kola
- Damiana
- Sarsparilla root
- Garlic
- Capsicum
- Chickweed

Herbal V by Smart Health USA, Inc. This blend is carried in many places, including a variety of large, nationwide health food stores. This product is marketed as "the all-natural alternative to prescription treatment" and also says that it is an "ultra pleasure delivery system." Men are to take "two tablets before romantic activity as a dietary supplement." Although the bottle never comes out and says what its for, well, we think it's rather easy to figure out at this point! Here is the list of herbal sex ingredients found in two tablets:
- Yohimbe extract, 250 mg
- Avena sativa extract, 150 mg
- Saw palmetto extract, 100 mg
- Guarana extract, 300 mg
- Siberian ginseng extract, 30 mg

Lady Herbal V by Smart Health USA, Inc. This product contains the same herbal combinations as Herbal V, though some are found in slightly different amounts, presumably to allow for differences between men's and women's body chemistry.

Other providers of a variety of herbal blends are listed below:
- Centrum
- One-A-Day

- Twin Lab (This company markets its products under many different names, including Alvita and Nature's Herbs.)
- Futurebiotics
- Irwin Naturals
- Nature's Sunshine
- Human Development Technology
- Nature's Fingerprint
- Nature's Way
- Vita-worth
- Nature Made
- Nature's Resource
- Schiff

This list is obviously not comprehensive, but examples are given just to provide an idea of how many companies are currently manufacturing and marketing herbal products. Most of these companies, as well as many others, make their products in single form as well as in various herbal combinations. Combination products are becoming increasingly more popular, and you'll find many similar herbs bundled together in these products. You can easily find yohimbe and damiana together, as well as blends of goldenseal and fo-ti.

Sex Herbs in Food Products

One of the latest trends is to consume herbs in the form of a nutrition bar or even in a drink. But be cautioned: Some of these products don't have enough herbs contained within them to do much good. Again, know the dosage you're looking for and read the label. In an herb shop or health food store, you'll probably find that the sales staff will know a lot about these products. Another consideration when choosing food products that contain sex herbs is their calorie level. Many of these products contain a substantial amount of calories and need to be dealt with by adjusting the rest of your calorie intake.

Nutrition Bars   Many nutrition bars are quite appealing in taste and are available in different flavors, such as chocolate, vanilla, and peanut butter. You'll probably even find an assortment on the shelf at the gym where you work out. One brand of nutrition bars, **Jolt,** contains numerous ingredients, including these sex herbs: guarana seed, ginkgo biloba, and panax ginseng. Again, no amounts of these herbs are listed, but hey, it only contains 4 grams of fat! Other brands may also add sex herbs to their energy or nutrition bars—take the time to read labels to discover which bars might work for you.

Herbal Beverages   The herbal drinks are the latest rage. They are prettily packaged, often in very colorful, eye-catching bottles. These herbal drinks usually have names that suggest what effects they might have on the drinker. However, they usually contain only a little of the active herb, and do not have to list specific amounts of herbal ingredients. Here are some of the most common herbal drinks available.

SoBe is perhaps the company with the widest range of herbal beverages. Here is a partial list:

- 3G teas, a series of teas (black, green, oolong, and red) that include the 3 Gs of ginseng, ginkgo, and guarana
- Powerline, which includes guarana, yohimbe, and arginine
- Wisdom drink, which includes St. John's Wort, gingko, and gotu kola
- Zen blend, which includes three forms of ginseng: Asian, Siberian, and American
- Eros drink, which includes damiana, fo-ti, and dong quai

Another popular brand you may find available in many stores is the **Arizona Tea Company.** Two of its current flavors include some sex herbs that you may benefit from:

- Arizona Herbal Tea with honey, which includes chamomile, gingko, ginseng extract, and licorice extract
- Green Tea with Ginseng and Plum Juice

Hansen's offers a beverage called d-stress formula. It contains a variety of vitamins, along with the herbs St. John's wort, kava, and chamomile. This brand actually—perhaps even bravely—lists the amounts of all of these ingredients on the label.

Herbal drinks these days aren't just packaged in flashy single-use bottles, but are also available in many stores in larger containers—and in more plainly packaged bottles or jugs. One such company is **Futurebiotics.** One of its drinks has no name in particular, but contains three forms of ginseng. **Langer's** also offers juice beverages with various herbs added, such as goldenseal and gingko.

Herbal teas also offer an easy way to obtain your sex herbs. **Celestial Seasonings** is a well-known, nationally distributed marketer of a range of teas containing a variety of herbs that can be helpful to sex. There are many other regional brands offering similar products.

Think of other, less-obvious places where you might find sex herbs as food ingredients, as well. For instance, cough drops often contain licorice. Candies often contain anise. Breath mints often contain peppermint. Again, amounts of these herbs contained in the products may be small, but it may be worth a few cents and a little extra effort to see if these food products work to help you improve your sex life.

* * *

The possibility for combinations of herbal products is almost endless—and even mindboggling at times. But by checking many sources, reading labels carefully, and talking with people knowledgeable about herbs, you are likely to find an herbal blend that can best meet your goal for enhancing your sex life.

Resources

Information About Herbs

Ask Dr. Weil (The Vitamin Shoppe)
web site: cgi.pathfinder.com/drweil

HealthWorld Online
web site: www.healthy.net

Herb Research Foundation
1007 Pearl Street, Suite 200
Boulder, CO 80302
phone: 800-748-2617
e-mail: info@herbs.org
web site: www.herbs.org

U.S. Food and Drug Administration
HFE-88
5600 Fishers Lane
Rockville, MD 20857
phone: 888-463-6332
web site: www.fda.gov

Resources for Herb Seeds

Companion Plants
7247 N. Coolville Ridge Road
Athens, OH 45701
phone: 740-593-3092
e-mail: complants@frognet.net
web site: www.frognet.net/companion_plants/

Dabney Herbs
P.O. Box 22061
Louisville, KY 40252-0061
phone: 502-893-5198
e-mail: Dabneyherb@win.net
web site: www.dabneyherbs.com

Desert Woman Botanicals
P.O. Box 263
Gila, NM 88038
phone: 505-535-2860

Elixir Farm Botanicals
General Delivery
Brixey, MO 65618
phone: 877-315-7333
e-mail: efb@aristotle.net
web site: www.elixirfarm.com

Goodwin Creek
P.O. Box 83
Williams, OR 97544
phone: 541-846-7357

Horizon Herbs
P.O. Box 69
Williams, OR 97544
phone: 541-846-6704
e-mail: herbseed@chatlink.com
web site: www.chatlink.com/~herbseed/

Johnny's Seeds
Rt. 1, Box 2580
Foss Hill Road
Albion, ME
phone: 207-437-9294
e-mail: commercial@johnnyseeds.com
web site: www.johnnyseeds.com

Sources for Buying Bulk Herbs

Frontier Cooperative Herbs
3021 78th Street
P.O. Box 299
Norway, IA 52318
phone: 800-669-3275
web site: www.frontierherb.com

Pacific Botanicals
4350 Fish Hatchery Road
Grants Pass, OR 97527
phone: 541-479-7777

Blessed Herbs
109 Barre Plains Road
Oakham, ME 01068
phone: 508-882-3839

Starwest Botanicals
11253 Trade Center Drive
Rancho Cordova, CA 95742
phone: 916-638-8100
web site: www.starwest_botanicals.com

Desert Woman Botanicals
P. O. Box 263
Gila, NM 88038
phone: 505-535-2860

Other Products

South Beach Beverage Company
phone: 1-800-588-0548
web site: www.sobebev.com

References

Ambrosino, Susan, and Ray, Daniel P. *The Incredible Healing Power of Herbs*. Lantana, Florida: Micromags, 1998.

The American Heritage Dictionary. 3d ed. New York: Dell Publishing, 1994.

Balch, M.D., James F., and Balch, C.N.C., Phyllis A. *Prescription for Nutritional Healing*. 2d ed. Garden City Park, New York: Avery Publishing Group, 1997.

Blakely, Tim, and Sturdinvant, Lee. *Medicinal Herbs in the Garden, Field and Marketplace*. Friday Harbor, Washington: San Juan Naturals, 1999.

Brinker, M.D., Francis. *Herb Contraindications and Drug Interactions*. Sandy, Oregon: Eclectic Institute, 1997.

Cameron, Myra. *Lifetime Encyclopedia of Natural Remedies*. West Nyack, New York: Parker Publishing, 1993.

Cortese, M.D., Bernard. *Perimenopause*. Freedom, California: Crossing Press, 1998.

Crawford, Amanda McQuade. *The Herbal Menopause Book*. Freedom, California: Crossing Press, 1996.

Duke, Ph.D., James. *The Green Pharmacy*. New York: St. Martin's, 1997.

Elkins, Rita. *The Complete Home Health Advisor*. Pleasant Grove, Utah: Woodland Health Books, 1994.

Evennett, Karen. *Garlic: The Natura Remedy*. Berkeley, California: Ulysses Press, 1998.

Fighting Disease. Emmaus, Pennsylvania: Rodale Books, 1995.

Krieger, Lisa M. Lousy sex life quite common, research finds. *San Jose Mercury News*, Feb. 10, 1999.

Leyel, C. F., ed. *A Modern Herbal*. New York: Barnes and Noble, 1996.

Merriam-Webster's Collegiate Dictionary. 10th ed. Springfield, Massachusetts: Merriam-Webster, 1997.

The Natural Guide to Medicinal Herbs and Plants. New York: Barnes and Noble, 1998.

Nickell, Nancy L. *Nature's Aphrodisiacs*. Freedom, California: Crossing Press, 1999.

Pierce, Andrea. *The American Pharmaceutical Association Practical Guide to Natural Medicines*. New York: Stonesong Press, William Morrow and Company, 1999.

Ritchason, M.D., Jack. *The Little Herb Encyclopedia*. Pleasant Grove, Utah: Woodland Health Books, 1995.

Rodale's Illustrated Encyclopedia of Herbs. Emmaus, Pennsylvania: Rodale Press, 1987.

St. Claire, Debra. *Pocket Herbal Reference Guide*. Freedom, California: Crossings Press, 1992.

Sunset Western Garden Book. Menlo Park, California: Sunset Publishing, 1995.

Index

Please note: Exact repeated mentions of specific conditions, effects, and problems are not indexed here.

Ulysses Press Health Books

A Natural Approach Books

Written in a friendly, nontechnical style, *A Natural Approach* books address specific health issues and show you how to take an active part in your own treatment. Believing that disease is more than a combination of symptoms, these books offer integrated mind/body programs that take a positive, preventative approach.

ANXIETY & DEPRESSION
ISBN 1-56975-118-8, 144 pp,
$9.95

CANDIDA
ISBN 1-56975-153-6, 208 pp,
$11.95

ENDOMETRIOSIS
ISBN 1-56975-088-2, 184 pp,
$9.95

FREE YOURSELF FROM
TRANQUILIZERS & SLEEPING PILLS
ISBN 1-56975-074-2, 192 pp,
$9.95

IRRITABLE BLADDER &
INCONTINENCE
ISBN 1-56975-089-0, 112 pp,
$8.95

IRRITABLE BOWEL SYNDROME
2nd edition, ISBN 1-56975-188-9,
256 pp, $13.95

MIGRAINES
ISBN 1-56975-140-4, 240 pp,
$10.95

PANIC ATTACKS
2nd edition, ISBN 1-56975-187-0,
144 pp, $9.95

Other Health Titles

THE ANCIENT AND HEALING ART OF AROMATHERAPY
ISBN 1-56975-094-7, 96 pp, $14.95
Discusses the benefits and history of aromatherapy.

THE ANCIENT AND HEALING ART OF CHINESE HERBALISM
ISBN 1-56975-139-0, 96 pp, $14.95
Offers a beautifully illustrated history and demonstrates the uses of Chinese herbalism.

THE BOOK OF KOMBUCHA
ISBN 1-56975-049-1, 160 pp, $11.95
Explains the benefits of and addresses concerns about Kombucha, the widely used Chinese "tea mushroom."

CIDER VINEGAR: THE NATURAL REMEDY
ISBN 1-56975-141-2, 144 pp, $8.95
Gives detailed information—not just hype—about the safe use of cider vinegar.

GARLIC: THE NATURAL REMEDY
ISBN 1-56975-097-1, 152 pp, $9.95
Provides a comprehensive look at the proven remedies of garlic.

HEALING REIKI: REUNITE MIND, BODY AND SPIRIT WITH HEALING ENERGY
ISBN 1-56975-162-5, 128 pp, $16.95
Examines the meaning, attitudes and history of Reiki while providing practical tips for receiving and giving this universal life energy.

HEPATITIS C: A PERSONAL GUIDE TO GOOD HEALTH
2nd edition, ISBN 1-56975-183-8, 180 pp, $13.95
Identifies the causes and symptoms of hepatitis C and presents conventional and alternative treatments for coping with the disease.

KNOW YOUR BODY: THE ATLAS OF ANATOMY
2nd edition, ISBN 1-56975-166-8, 160 pp, $12.95
Provides a a comprehensive, full-color guide to the human body.

MOOD FOODS
ISBN 1-56975-023-8, 192 pp, $11.95
Shows how the foods you eat influence your emotions and behavior.

NEW AGAIN!: THE 28-DAY DETOX PLAN FOR BODY AND SOUL
ISBN 1-56975-190-0, 128 pp, $16.95
Allows you to free your body *and* mind from toxins and live a healthy and balanced life.

THE 7 HEALING CHAKRAS: UNLOCKING YOUR BODY'S ENERGY CENTERS
ISBN 1-56975-168-4, 240 pp, $14.95
Explores the essence of chakras, vortices of energy that connect the physical body with the spiritual.

YOUR NATURAL PREGNANCY: A GUIDE TO COMPLEMENTARY THERAPIES
ISBN 1-56975-059-9, 240 pp, $16.95
Details alternative therapies ranging from aromatherapy to yoga that can benefit pregnant women.

———

To order these books call 800-377-2542 or 510-601-8301, fax 510-601-8307, e-mail ulysses@ulyssespress.com, or write to Ulysses Press, P.O. Box 3440, Berkeley, CA 94703-3440. All retail orders are shipped free of charge. California residents must include sales tax. Allow two to three weeks for delivery.

Beth Ann Petro Roybal, M.A. and Gayle L. Skowronski have collaborated on many patient education projects over the years.

Beth Roybal is an award-winning writer, editor, and instructional designer of books, brochures, videos, and computer-based programs dealing with health and safety topics. She, her husband, and their two toddlers spend free time hiking the coastal Central California hills and tending an orchard and garden at their hillside home overlooking California's Pajaro Valley.

Gayle Skowronski has worked at a range of jobs within the health care industry. She has put her inside knowledge of this field to work in researching and writing materials for patient and public education. Her two teenage daughters are budding writers themselves, providing editorial opinions while Gayle and her husband shuttle them to their various activities around the Clearwater area on Florida's Gulf Coast.